Treating Psoriasis with Chinese Herbal Medicine

of related interest

Healing Brain Injury with Chinese Medical Approaches
Integrative Approaches for Practitioners
Douglas S. Wingate
ISBN 978 1 84819 402 1
eISBN 978 0 85701 356 9

Cosmetic Acupuncture, Second Edition
A Traditional Chinese Medicine Approach to Cosmetic and Dermatological Problems
Radha Thambirajah
ISBN 978 1 84819 267 6
eISBN 978 0 85701 215 9

Facial Enhancement Acupuncture
Clinical Use and Application
Paul Adkins
Illustrated by Roger Dutton
ISBN 978 1 84819 129 7
eISBN 978 0 85701 103 9

Treating Emotional Trauma with Chinese Medicine
Integrated Diagnostic and Treatment Strategies
CT Holman, M.S., L.Ac.
ISBN 978 1 84819 318 5
eISBN 978 0 85701 271 5

The Art and Practice of Diagnosis in Chinese Medicine
Nigel Ching
ISBN 978 1 84819 314 7
eISBN 978 0 85701 267 8

Treating Psoriasis with Chinese Herbal Medicine

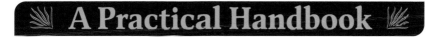
A Practical Handbook

Revised Edition

Sabine Schmitz

Foreword by Steve Clavey

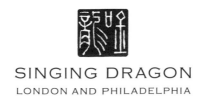

SINGING DRAGON

LONDON AND PHILADELPHIA

First published by Chinamed-Publishing, Cologne, Germany, 2018

This revised edition first published in 2020
by Singing Dragon
an imprint of Jessica Kingsley Publishers
73 Collier Street
London N1 9BE, UK
and
400 Market Street, Suite 400
Philadelphia, PA 19106, USA

www.singingdragon.com

Library of Congress Cataloging in Publication Data
A CIP catalog record for this book is available from the Library of Congress

British Library Cataloguing in Publication Data
A CIP catalogue record for this book is available from the British Library

ISBN 978 1 78775 349 5
eISBN 978 1 78775 350 1

Printed and bound in China

Dedicated to my teacher, Professor Mǎ Lìlì 马丽俐.
I will always appreciate your knowledge and generosity.

Appreciating human life, appreciating good health!

Contents

Foreword

WE ALL HAVE skin in the game.

But the game, despite what some say, is not only about boundaries and borders and protection from the outside world, it is also about free passage between realms, a balancing of pressures, a sensing, of contact, and, more importantly, of touch.

In fact some of the wisest amongst us say that all these demarcations are illusory, there is no "inside" or "outside" world, it is all one thing in flux, with temporary expedient separations that dissolve and reform as the need arises. It was none other than Ludwig Feuerbach who said "Being-in-the-body means being-in-the-world. So many senses—so many pores. The self is nothing other than the *porous* self."[1]

But when that boundary goes wrong there can be problems. Take, for example, the idea that it needs to be thicker, stronger, tougher, that resources need to be sent to certain sections to reinforce the wall against the outside world. Things heat up. Imbalances occur, then proliferate. Violence can begin, breakdown result: cracks appear, blood is shed.

And this idea need not be due to actual external impacts, but can occur from a perception that things are not as they should be, of disquiet, of stress; negative emotions that trigger an insane race to toughen up the defenses.

That is what happens in psoriasis, a vicious cycle of hyper-proliferation of keratinocytes in the epidermis. None of the Western conventional treatments to date have done other than try to suppress the symptoms, and suppression, if it works at all, does so only for a limited time.

Chinese medicine has a different approach: look for the root cause, the underlying imbalance, and work to redress that. When the violence at the surface is extreme, and suppression measures such as corticosteroids have been used, it may be necessary to continue them for a short while, but the goal is always to lessen the source of the problem to achieve a lasting result.

This book presents a focused and in-depth treatment of the psoriatic condition, including its many variations and further consequences, such as psoriatic arthritis. The author has gone out of her way to provide well over 50 color photos of skin lesions with crucial points of differentiation illustrated, and over 40 color photos of tongue types linked to pattern differentiation. Some of my favorite aspects of this work by Dr. Schmitz are the nine examples of pattern differentiation and particularly the herb couplets that speak of deep experience, and the directions for preparing the various ointments, creams, lotions, and washes that can be so helpful for patients.

May you find it as useful a tool for restoring balance at the boundaries as I have.

Steve Clavey
Melbourne

Endnote

1   Some Comments on the "Beginning of Philosophy" of Dr. J.F. Reiff, 1841.

Acknowledgments

A SPECIAL THANK YOU to Steve Clavey for his generosity in reviewing my manuscript and providing useful suggestions. I would like to thank my former tutor, Professor Mǎ Lìlì. Without her knowledge and expertise, my work in Chinese dermatology would certainly not be the same. Fāng Yīmiào, my former classmate, and Yáng Zǐ, my patient translator, deserve recognition for their generous and continuous support in the collection of patient data and translations from Chinese to English (and vice versa) during my studies and afterwards. I would also like to recognize Karin Hirmer, my thorough English proofreader. And further thanks to Mary-Jo Bevin for conscientiously proofreading my manuscript. Finally, I offer my gratitude to Claire Wilson from Singing Dragon for believing in this book and the idea it stands for. Your support is highly appreciated. But mostly I would like to thank my husband, Hans, for his support and understanding in times when I did not have much time.

Disclaimer

THE INFORMATION in this book is given to the best of the author's knowledge. However, the author cannot be held responsible for any error or omission. The author disclaims any responsibility for any injury and/or damage to persons or property in connection with the use of the material contained in this book. Chinese medicine is professional medicine and this is a specialist book. The author does not advocate or endorse self-medication by laypersons. Laypersons interested in availing themselves of the treatment described in this book are advised to seek out a qualified professional practitioner of Chinese medicine. It is the responsibility of the treating physician to determine the method, the dosages of each therapeutic drug, and duration of treatment for the patient.

About the Author

SABINE SCHMITZ (M. Med. TCM) is a graduate of the Zhèjiāng Chinese Medical University in Hángzhōu, China, where she majored in Chinese medical dermatology. Her vast treasures of knowledge from China and her many years of experience benefit numerous patients with chronic and complex skin diseases, as well as many patients with other diseases.

Earlier in her career, Sabine worked in hospitals, laboratories, universities, and national and international clinical research for 15 years. Sabine is based in Cologne, Germany, and has a busy Traditional Chinese Medicine (TCM) practice specializing in skin diseases, gynecological disorders, and infertility treatment. She mainly works with Chinese herbal medicine and acupuncture.

Preface

MY MOTIVES for writing this book are manifold. When I studied in China, I acquired a very good overview of the information and literature available on the subject of psoriasis and of the latest research. Thus, the main reason for writing this book is that, at present, literature about the application of Chinese medicine in the treatment of psoriasis is rare, is scattered in different places, or lacks depth and scope in methods and explanations. I found this to be true when I compiled a very detailed literature review for my master's degree in China, with my key subject being Chinese dermatology, in particular psoriasis. However, while performing this initial literature research, I found hardly any books in English that sufficiently address the application of Chinese medicine in treating psoriasis. There are only three books on the market in English that deal with psoriasis.[1] Two of them only assign one chapter to this skin disease. The third one[2] is no longer in print.[3] It is neither well produced nor helpful, and lacks focus as it dwells on all kinds of treatments without structure. Additionally, the results presented in various articles on psoriasis available in English[4] are redundant. All in all, I can only point out the insufficient state of literature regarding this topic, and note that this unsatisfactory documentation deviates from the analysis and treatment of psoriasis that I have observed and followed in my practice and during my studies in China. This is why I am convinced that a detailed written account of the analysis and treatment practice in TCM has been long overdue—an account that includes the adaptations to our modern context, and the integration of knowledge gained in past decades.

Chinese herbal medicine has been used to treat psoriasis since ancient times. The earliest ancient description of psoriasis from a TCM perspective can be found in a book from the Suí Dynasty,[5] called *Zhū Bìng Yuán Hóu Lùn* (General Treatise on the Etiology and Symptomology of Diseases), by Cháo Yuánfāng. Yet societies and their lifestyles have changed. In our more stressful and challenging times, chronic skin diseases like psoriasis seem to be increasing. Living conditions have changed and we, as TCM doctors, need to take the patients' emotions and environment into account. It would be a mistake not to do this—to not consider the obvious, which is often the root cause of the disease. Emotional changes, especially "inappropriate" or excessive emotions, play an important role in the onset of psoriasis. The Liver (*gān* 肝)[6] plays a crucial role in treating psoriasis in cases of emotional changes. Interestingly, TCM books discussing psoriasis very often miss one of the most common TCM syndromes occurring nowadays, which is Liver qì stagnation syndrome with excess heat. This book, among other things, describes the mechanism behind the pattern of Liver qì stagnation (*gān qì yù jié* 肝气郁结) and the resulting negative impact on the skin, and it details the corresponding treatment. Furthermore, it explores the most common TCM syndromes in depth. Finally, aspects of my own clinical experience are included to fill out and bring to life the theory in this book.

Moreover, this book also presents the latest research findings about Chinese herbs commonly used and most effective with regard to the modern pharmacological mode of action in the treatment of psoriasis. Chapter 5 details other essential and useful herbs that I use in my clinic and, perhaps more importantly, lists the formulas that have been proved to be most effective and have not been mentioned in this context before.

In order to treat patients successfully, we cannot simply look at efficacy but also need to consider patients' safety. What use is it if a treatment seems to be effective in improving affected skin areas but the patient experiences significant side effects? In the course of my studies on psoriasis in China, we performed a case series with 56 patients to prove the efficacy and safety of Chinese herbal medicine in the treatment of psoriasis. With the background of all clinical data collected and from my personal clinical experience in treating patients with skin diseases, it is evident that TCM offers a safe and effective treatment option for psoriasis, based on natural sources, and with fewer adverse effects. My clinical experience confirms the high efficacy and low recurrence that TCM offers, along with a variety of treatment methods and flexibility in the use of herbs. This—and the fact that TCM has few side effects—make it a promising alternative therapy to conventional medicine.

I am glad to share my findings and considerations with all readers of this book. This book marks the beginning of a series of handbooks on Chinese dermatology. I hope that this and all upcoming publications will serve as a useful resource for the treatment of patients with complex skin diseases in everyday practice.

Endnotes

1 Xu, Y. (2004) *Dermatology in Traditional Chinese Medicine* (1st edition). St Albans: Donica Publishing Ltd. Lu, C.J. and Xuan, G.W. (2008) *The Clinical Practice of Chinese Medicine: Psoriasis and Cutaneous Pruritis*. Beijing: People's Medical Publishing House. Li Lin (1990) *Treatment of Psoriasis with Traditional Chinese Medicine* (1st edition). Hong Kong: Hai Feng Publishing

2 Li Lin (1990) *Treatment of Psoriasis with Traditional Chinese Medicine* (1st edition). Hong Kong: Hai Feng Publishing.

3 In order to know what I am talking about, I made a long journey to buy this book from a secondhand bookshop in Holland.

4 For example: Lu, C.J., Yu, J.J., and Deng, J.W. (2012) "Disease-syndrome combination clinical study of psoriasis: Present status, advantages, and prospects." *Chinese Journal of Integrative Medicine 18*, 3, 166–171; or Tse, T.W. (2003) "Use of common Chinese herbs in the treatment of psoriasis." *Clinical and Experimental Dermatology 28*, 5, 469–475.

5 Suí Dynasty (581–618 AD).

6 *Pīnyīn* will be given first for all Chinese terms throughout the book, then Chinese. This should make it more accessible for all those who do not speak Chinese.

Introduction

Psoriasis (*bái bǐ* 白疕, or in common usage *niú pí xuǎn* 牛皮癣) is a recurring, chronic inflammatory skin disease, characterized by thick, dry, and silver-colored scaly plaques. Although it primarily affects the skin and nails, the joints can also be involved. The etiology is not clear, but it is linked to genetic and immune system abnormalities, resulting in hyperproliferation of the epidermis and inflammation of the skin.

Western medicine does not offer any complete cure for psoriasis at present. The various treatments currently available only aim at reducing the intensity of its symptoms. The current treatments range from external (topical) application to internal (systemic) therapy as well as UV phototherapy. These treatments are often burdensome, unpleasant, and largely unsatisfactory. Oral medication is usually reserved for severe cases because of potential side effects. The intake of oral methotrexate (MTX) or retinoic acid (marketed as Roaccutane), for instance, may adversely impact the patient's physical and mental health. External use of ointments, which contain ingredients such as glucocorticoids, have shown poor efficacy after the discontinuation of skin treatment: recurrence and aggravation have been observed. Therefore, patients become frustrated and start looking for alternative treatment options.

An additional factor in the frustration with Western medicine is that patients nowadays are better informed than they used to be. Awareness concerning pharmaceutical products has changed significantly, with regard not only to their efficacy but also to the benefits versus the risks of the drugs prescribed. For Western psoriasis patients, therefore, a suitable therapy proven to be without recurrence and aggravation has yet to be found. This is what TCM can offer. When the advantages of TCM are explained in a simple and clear manner, patients are quite open to taking new paths and trying new approaches.

In China, TCM is a popular method to treat this disease, because the positive results are known. It is fascinating to consider how long TCM has been used for the treatment of psoriasis in China: over one thousand years. And this only refers to specialist treatments of dermatological diseases, such as psoriasis. TCM in general can produce records for more than two thousand years of medical development. In comparison, the origins of empirical conventional medicine barely stretch to three hundred years. This is something that should be stressed to patients who consult a TCM doctor for the first time. Without exaggeration, it can be stated that TCM offers a variety of internal and external treatment methods that allow for a flexible approach in the use of remedies. This flexibility is essential to the treatment of skin diseases, because the tendency of skin diseases is to develop and change rapidly. This variation has to be reflected in their medical treatment, which needs to be flexible and applicable. Monitoring and checking the patient's progress continuously is thus crucial. Practice shows that even a minor external or emotional irritant can worsen a skin condition that seemed to be perfectly fine the previous day.

Finally, Chinese herbal therapies–the focus of this book–are not only effective but also safe. Patients generally comply well, and the remission period seems to be longer lasting compared with conventional medicine.

The occurrence of psoriasis is increasing, although the reasons for this upsurge have not been identified.[1] Considering that the worldwide prevalence of psoriasis is around 2%[2] and rising, it seems obvious that there is a definite demand and need for more specialist literature exploring this area of TCM. This book reviews the long history of Chinese medical dermatology and explains psoriasis from a TCM perspective. It depicts the most common TCM syndromes and introduces the corresponding internal and external treatments for each case. Lifestyle suggestions are presented, as they are crucial to the patient's recovery–keeping in mind that the patient him- or herself is always a part of the treatment. Finally, clinical cases are explained and the latest biochemical research results are taken into account.

Having learned, applied, and experienced the advantages of Chinese treatment options, it is quite obvious that TCM offers the most beneficial treatment for patients suffering from this chronic disease. By choosing the most suitable treatment method and knowing the effects, TCM provides immense flexibility in treatment options and a broad range of applications. This is essential since not all patients with the same Western medicine diagnosis can or should be treated in the same way. In psoriasis, for example, TCM allows for individual treatment, fully adapted to each individual's needs, because it takes into account different locations, different stages, and different sub-types according to their appearance.

Endnotes

1 Icen, M., Crowson, C.S., McEvoy, M.T., Dann, F.J., Gabriel, S.E., and Maradit Kremers, H. (2009) "Trends in incidence of adult-onset psoriasis over three decades: A population-based study." *Journal of the American Academy of Dermatology 60*, 3, 394–401.

2 World Health Organization (2013) *Psoriasis: Report by the Secretariat,* EB133/5. Geneva: WHO.

1

Overview and Basics of Chinese Dermatology

IT IS ASSUMED that the reader is familiar with TCM foundations. The information on the basics of TCM dermatology is primarily aimed at TCM students and beginners. Experts can, of course, skip this chapter. Nonetheless, the information compiled in this chapter can be a valuable resource and refresher for everyone, TCM dermatologists, general TCM doctors, or students of TCM.

An Overview of the History of Chinese Medical Dermatology (*Pí Fū Kē* 皮肤科)

Chinese medical dermatology can refer back to many centuries of experience, with detailed records of the effects of Chinese herbs and acupuncture on the condition of the skin. Comprehensive descriptions of the treatment of specific skin diseases were put down in writing by ancient scholars, and their clinical histories and notes offer a depth of experience we still utilize today in our practice.

Yet time does not stand still. A great deal of research into Chinese medicine has been conducted both inside and outside of China. In addition to clinical studies, official monographs about almost every Chinese medical plant are available at the European Medicines Agency (EMEA) and the World Health Organization (WHO). These monographs present a detailed introduction and provide a scientific overview on the safety, efficacy, and quality control of commonly used medicinal plants in Chinese dermatology. Moreover, gathered information about chemical compositions, pharmacological effects, toxicology, clinical studies, and research has been incorporated into the different textbooks of *materia medica* which are used by TCM doctors worldwide.[1]

The result of this combination of a rich history and modern developments is an independent and sophisticated specialty in Chinese medicine, which can be effectively employed in the treatment of many, if not most, skin diseases. This is particularly true for the most common skin problems presenting in our clinics, where the effectiveness of conventional medicine therapy is very poor. Psoriasis is a very good example of this.

Developmental Changes in Chinese Dermatology

In ancient China, Chinese dermatology was a part of the general category *wài kē* 外科. Medical fields such as traumatology and surgery were also classified as a part of *wài kē* at that time. *Wài* refers to the outside of the body and comprises the skin, hair, muscles, flesh, sinews, and bones. The term *kē* means subject, branch, or field. *Wài kē*, or "external medicine," refers to the diagnosis and treatment of conditions on the exterior of the body. This includes skin conditions such as sores and abscesses, and diseases of the eye, ear, nose, and mouth. In contrast, *nèi kē* 内科 (internal medicine) refers to diseases occurring inside the body and the *nèi*, or the inside, comprising the viscera and bowels. Chinese dermatology was recognized much later in history as a separate specialty in TCM.

The following presents a short overview on the publication history in Chinese dermatology.

Early classical literature	Small sections dedicated to Chinese dermatology (*pí fū kē*)	<ul><li>Many important doctors devoted to the study and practice of external medicine</li><li>References to external medicine scattered in medical textbooks</li><li>No independent section of medical literature</li></ul>
Sòng Dynasty[2] 1263	*Wài Kē Jīng Yào* (Essence of Diagnosis and Treatment of External Diseases) by Chén Zìmíng	<ul><li>First book solely focused on *wài kē*</li><li>Establishment of external medicine and traumatic surgery as independent branches of Chinese medicine</li><li>Particularization of the medical necessity of medical measures in surgery</li></ul>
Yuán Dynasty[3] 1335	*Wài Kē Jīng Yì* (Treatment of Surgical Diseases) by Qí Dézhī	<ul><li>Compilation of the medical knowledge of external diseases prior to the Yuán Dynasty</li><li>Treatment of external diseases should start with regulating body's internal system considering pathogenic factors</li><li>External disease arises from disharmony between yīn 阴 and yáng 阳, or stagnating qì 气 and xuè 血</li><li>Creation of new therapies, e.g. wet compresses and methods for draining pus</li></ul>

Míng Dynasty[4]	Wāng Jī (1463–1539)	▪ Medical writer and clinical practitioner from Ānhuī Province south of Nánjīng
1531	*Wài Kē Lǐ Lì* (Exemplars for Applying the Principles of External Medicine)	▪ Preface: "external medicine [i.e. surgery] deals with ulcers, abscesses, sores and boils…seen on the exterior" ▪ Wāng Jī's views on *wài kē*: "surgical" doctors[5] do not perform invasive surgery associated with today ▪ All external manifestations of illness have internal root ▪ Emphasized the combination of internal treatments, e.g. herbal decoctions, and external treatments, e.g. ointments, washes, acupuncture, or moxibustion ▪ Vast number of case histories
1522–1633	*Wāng Shíshān Yī Shū Bā Zhǒng* (Eight Medical Books of Stone Mountain Wang) One book of this compilation is *Shí Shān Yī Àn* (Medical Cases of Wāng Jī)	▪ Numerous cases of *wài kē* section, e.g. itchy body, foot sores and breast lumps[6] ▪ More than one hundred of Wāng Jī's medical cases (collected by his students)
Míng and Qīng[7] Dynasties		▪ Chinese dermatology flourished with the publication of several works that presented external diseases
1604, late Míng Dynasty	*Wài Kē Qǐ Xuán* (Profound Insights on External Diseases) by Shēn Dǒuyuán	▪ Consisting of 12 volumes ▪ Considered China's first atlas of skin diseases ▪ Contains about 200 different diseases and treatments
1617	*Wài Kē Zhèng Zōng* (True Lineage of External Medicine) by Chén Shígōng	▪ New therapeutic recommendations for skin diseases, including ointments ▪ Summary of medical achievements before the Míng Dynasty ▪ Diagnoses, therapies, medical records and prescriptions ▪ Precise surgical procedures, e.g. removal of nasal polyps,[8] trachelorrhaphy, and cancer therapies
1665	*Wài Kē Dà Chéng* (Great Compendium of External Medicine) by Qí Kūn	▪ Chinese dermatology became increasingly sophisticated and numerous specialist books were published

1740	One book of this compilation is *Shí Shān Yī Àn* (Medical Cases of Wāng Jī)	▪ More than one hundred of Wāng Jī's medical cases (collected by his students)
1831	*Wài Kē Zhèng Zhì Quán Shū* (Complete Book of Patterns and Treatments in External Medicine) by Xǔ Kèchāng	

▪ Most classics on external diseases and treatments reprinted in modern times
▪ New dermatological textbooks
▪ Some available in English

The Daily Routine in Chinese Medical Dermatology

Dermatology is one of the most difficult areas in TCM. The disease patterns are complex, and so many skin diseases are deep-rooted and resistant to treatment. The challenge of diagnosing and treating skin diseases requires a highly skilled ability to observe and to analyze. Every student of Chinese medicine soon finds that the knowledge one acquires from one's teachers cannot simply be imitated in clinic: imitation will not work; you must use your teacher's knowledge as a basis to build your own expertise. There are some factors that cannot be adapted, such as environmental circumstances or emotional and cultural factors. No matter how much experience you have gained throughout the years, the continuing process of learning from experienced teachers enables you to deepen both theoretical and practical understanding, learning refinements that improve your practice and prevent mistakes in application. This is the only way to deepen expertise and refine knowledge—an experience that will serve your patients as well.

A constant challenge in daily practice is that disease patterns often overlap. It is also important to note that most patients who come into a TCM practice have a long history of visiting allopathic skin specialists and have already tried multiple therapies. Again, most cases present not only with a skin disorder but also with other factors such as digestive or emotional issues. This is why patience is required from both the doctor and the patient over the course of the treatment. Patients need to be made aware of the fact that long-term conditions will take much longer to treat than conditions with a more recent onset.

Chinese dermatology deals with profound processes that manifest on the body's surface—the skin. Skin diseases must be understood in the context of the entire body, a perspective which is fundamentally different from conventional medicine. Diseases are considered through complex patterns of signs and symptoms that define each individual clinical presentation. In TCM, the goal is always to treat the pattern, which is regarded as the root cause. In other words, a purely symptom-based treatment as is frequently employed in conventional Western dermatology will not reach such a long-lasting resolution.

The initial diagnosis of the skin disease leaves us with multiple options for internal and external treatments. The following presents a step-by-step assessment of this process.

For a correct diagnosis of skin diseases according to TCM, it is essential to consider the following factors:

- an examination of the skin lesion (its onset, duration, location, appearance, and temperature)

- the exacerbating or relieving factors

- all associated symptoms such as itching, burning, scaling, bleeding, or discharge.

The focus in Chinese dermatology is always the skin lesion with all its presenting characteristics. This is clearly one of the most beneficial aspects in Chinese dermatology. Besides the presenting skin disease, factors such as emotions, sleep, diet, digestion, lifestyle, and environment (potential stress, overwork, night shifts), and the menstrual cycle in female patients, are important aspects of the Chinese diagnostic process. Moreover, by taking the pulse and tongue diagnosis into consideration, the therapist gathers information on how the body works as a whole. Then, once the Chinese diagnosis has been established, an individual treatment plan is created.

In severe or long-lasting skin diseases, Chinese herbs can be prescribed for both internal treatment and external application. One issue is important but often overlooked: in particularly stubborn cases it is often advisable to enquire after diet, living circumstances, and lifestyle habits. This is especially true for those patients with a chronic skin disease who expect instant results, or patients who state that they have already tried every method available. Practitioners might be surprised by what they will learn about bad eating habits, massive alcohol consumption, or a constant lack of sleep. For those patients it is essential to provide dietary advice and to explain what role their own behavior plays in maintaining their disease. Telling them to go to bed early or to reduce their workload to lessen stress may seem to be simple and obvious advice, but patients often find it hard to break habits. One approach is to help the patient understand that they are doing it for themselves. If you can help a patient realize that they are a part of the therapeutic process, substantial progress can be made.

Chinese Herbal Treatment Options in Chinese Medical Dermatology

The wide variety of treatment options developed over the centuries and the extensive range of internal and external applications TCM offers are a direct response to the flexibility required in curing complex disease patterns.

This section offers a general overview of commonly used internal and external treatment options in Chinese medical dermatology. Advantages and disadvantages of the available applications will be explained, and examples are listed by way of illustration. All of this is part of basic Chinese medicine education, but it can be helpful to explain it to the patient and can serve as an overview for students and beginners. A brief outline of specific external treatment options for psoriasis can be found in Appendix I.

Decoctions (*Jiān Jì* 煎剂)

Decoctions, or teas, of raw herbs are the most effective form of treatment. Herbal decoctions are prepared in three steps: first soaking, which allows the cell walls of the medicinal substance to expand for better extraction during boiling; then boiling in a ceramic pot (a ceramic pot is usually the best choice, because herbs like *ē jiāo* or *hé shǒu wū* are not suitable for being cooked in a metal pot); and lastly straining. The patient then drinks the strained liquid. To obtain the highest efficacy of the herbs when brewing, the herbs are usually boiled twice. Some herbs are added early, some later; some herbs are bagged and others are dissolved in water and taken directly without boiling.

Each prescription combines individual medicinal herbs selected in each case to fulfill the individual's needs. Decoctions are flexible in their application and allow easy adaptation of the prescription to the condition as it presents on a particular day. Thus, the patient will obtain an individually tailored prescription fitting his or her medical condition and current situation. One single pill can never be effective for thousands of patients, as seen in conventional medicine, when every one of these people has their own individual symptoms and different situation in life.

The substances gained from the use of a freshly brewed decoction are the most effective. Raw herbs can also be modified through processing techniques, known as *páo zhì* 炮制. *Páo zhì* is a traditional preparation process, which changes and specifies the therapeutic effect of medicinal plants. It reduces toxicity and unwanted side effects, changes pharmacological properties, enhances the precision of therapeutic effects, and changes the smell and taste of the plants. There are different preparation methods, such as roasting, frying, steaming, baking, calcinating, germinating, fermenting, or cooking individually or in special combinations. Applied in daily practice, that means that if you want to change the action—for example, strengthen a certain effect of an herb—or you want to make it more tolerable for patients with a weak digestion, then you can use *páo zhì*, depending on your needs. Any qualified TCM pharmacy is able to prepare it.

Another advantage of herbal decoctions is that the ingredients can be cooked for different lengths of time. Flowers, for example, are very light in nature and should only be cooked for a few minutes. Heavy substances such as minerals should be cooked for a longer time, at least 60 minutes, and they are often pre-cooked for this reason. In general, a fresh herbal decoction with a long cooking time is best for deep-rooted processes because it can reach the deep layers of the body and quickly attack the disease. This means that the correct location of the disease must be taken into account in order to cure illness. For external applications, herbs are only very briefly boiled because the effects must reach the surface.

In sum, within a complex and individual tailored herbal formula, many chemical reactions occur between the active ingredients of each single herb. The dosages of decoctions can be used with precision. A decoction can be modified in many ways and works fast. Additionally, in the West raw herbs are considerably cheaper than other application forms such as herbal granules.

Considering all this, when treating a serious case, raw herbs are always recommended. Although herbal decoctions do not taste good, patients usually tolerate them once the benefits are explained. Herbal decoctions are usually the best choice to treat difficult skin conditions. This can be seen when patients who have had good results taking raw herbs switch to granules—because of traveling, for instance. Regardless, if the same composition is given to the same patient, the difference is quite often distinct. Lesions return, they itch more, or they get redder.

Granules (*Kē Lì Jì* 颗粒剂) and Pills (*Piàn Jì* 片剂)

Granules are Chinese medicinal herbs extracted and compressed into granules by using modernized extraction and concentration technologies to replicate the traditional method of preparing medicinal decoction. In pills, the extracts are further processed and pressed into pill form for ease of consumption.

As granules and pills are not given in a fresh form, fillers such as cellulose and carrier substances such as lactose are added. Although there are no significant pharmacological, toxicological, and clinical studies to demonstrate the equivalence with decoctions,[9] it can be seen in clinical practice that granules are less effective as symptoms return and conditions worsen when patients switch to granules. Moreover, it seems quite difficult to determine the exact ratio of the herb available in the granule. The industry mentions several yield ratios–that is, the amount of product yielded from the extraction process. The standard yield ratio seems to be 5:1,[10] but the industry often just does not publish the exact ratio because yields can differ depending on factors such as whether the herbs (especially roots and fruits/seeds) are ground into smaller pieces, the length of extraction time, the solubility of the herb's ingredients in water, whether organic solvents are used, the pH of the extract solution, whether a temperature gradient is used, and the seasonality of the herb.[11] It also needs to be questioned which size of measuring spoon is used by patients. As a consequence of all of these factors, determining how to properly dose granules can be very difficult or almost impossible. Furthermore, for granules neither *páo zhì* nor different cooking time options are available. Simple practical disadvantages of granules are that they often clump together, they do not taste better than herbal decoctions, and they are usually more expensive than raw herbs.

However, granules are convenient and helpful in some situations, and better than no remedy–for instance, during travel, in circumstances where refrigeration is not available, or in situations where the patient does not want to or cannot drink decoctions, such as during pregnancy or after having taken decoctions for a long time. However, patients often come back after they have taken granules during travel and ask for herbal decoctions.

Tinctures (*Dīng Jì* 酊剂)

Tinctures are herbal preparations made in alcoholic bases. Tinctures are called medicinal liquor in Chinese, and they can be used internally or applied topically. A very commonly used dermatological tincture is, for example, a medicinal tincture made of *bǔ gǔ zhī* (*bǔ gǔ zhī dīng*). *Bǔ gǔ zhī* naturally contains psoralen, a parent compound in a family of natural products known as furocoumarins. Psoralen is known for its effect of increasing photosensitivity. This means that psoralen sensitizes the skin to sunlight and ultraviolet (UV) radiation. In psoriasis, *bǔ gǔ zhī* tincture can also be used topically. Psoralen intercalates into the DNA, and on exposure to UVA radiation it can form substances that induce apoptosis.[12] If the uncontrolled cell proliferation that is seen in the pathomechanism of psoriasis is stopped, the pathological formation of scales will be impeded. The therapeutic and photosensitizing actions of *bǔ gǔ zhī* are also frequently used in the treatment of vitiligo. As a phototoxic response after topical application, the melanocytes will be stimulated to produce more pigment. The white, non-pigmented spots become dark again—that is, re-pigmentation takes place.

Patients should be advised that they need to be very careful with external applications because tinctures greatly increase skin sensitivity. Therefore, they should be wary of long-term sun exposure, which can cause extreme skin reactions such as sunburn or irritation of previously injured or damaged skin areas. Incidentally, it must be also pointed out that a side effect of PUVA (psoralen + UVA) treatment is a higher risk of skin cancer.[13]

Taken internally, the use of herbal tinctures is not so common, but it can be a good interim solution in times where the patient does not drink herbal tea. For example, patients are commonly advised to drink one bag of Chinese herbal tea per week in less severe conditions. One bag of tea does not usually last the whole week, and so for the remaining days of the week the patient should take the tincture to support the effect of the raw herbs.

Washes (*Xǐ Dí* 洗涤) and Wet Compresses (*Shī Fū* 湿敷)

Herbal washes which are applied topically directly to the skin lesion can help with various types of skin problems such as itching, heat, inflammation, pustules, swellings, and ulcerations, and promotes healing of the skin. Herbal washes can be used as an external wash or as local wet compresses. For wet compresses, a folded piece of material, bandage, or small towel is immersed into a herbal decoction and then placed over the affected area for a certain period of time.

Special herbal combinations are known to have a disinfecting effect, such as *Sān Huáng Xǐ Jì*, made of *huáng bǎi*, *huáng qín*, *dà huáng*, and *kǔ shēn*. Because "yellow" (*huáng* in Chinese) is part of three of these four herb names, the formula is called "Three Yellow Cleanser Formula." This ancient topical formula is known for its effects of clearing heat, stopping itching, and arresting secretion, and it is often used in skin conditions such as acne, dermatitis, eczema, furuncles, and boils. One other example for a very simple herbal wash, which is very often prescribed for acne relief, is a herbal wash consisting only of *zhāng nǎo* (camphor). Very good results seem to have been relieving pain, swelling, and irritation in deep and painful pimples. But it has to be used with caution because *zhāng nǎo* is suitable for external application only. Patients should be informed that it is toxic if taken internally!

Herbal washes or wet compresses and also baths are mainly used in skin conditions that involve discharge. This method still allows the secretion of pathogenic fluids and pus while relieving heat, inflammation, pustules, or swellings. During acute stages, washes, compresses, and baths in particular should be taken with caution because of the potential risk of secondary inflammation. This can occur during the acute stage, when skin injuries or discharge can be present. Usually, wounds are exposed to some level of contamination, which does not necessarily lead to infection. However, a critical presence of bacteria—when the concentration of pathogenic microorganisms exceeds a tolerable level for normal skin healing—can allow bacteria to penetrate the skin, causing infection and impeding healing. Bacteria not only adhere to the skin lesion but can also remain present on medical equipment, bath surfaces, and medicinals added to the bath. In psoriasis, also remember that patients who have undergone therapy with immunosuppressives are at a significantly higher risk for getting an infection. This therapy can possibly be too intense or strong for these patients, due to very hot water. Moreover, crusts can open during drying and easily inflame. As with any other treatment modality, we must therefore weigh the use of therapy time and effort against objective evidence that supports its use for skin improvement in patients with psoriasis at the acute stage. This especially applies to medicinal baths. At a later stage, usually ointments and creams are used.

In summary, since the light texture of herbal decoctions offers a non-occluding effect, this method is able to heal the skin on a deeper level. A cream, for example, would enclose the discharge, and instead of pathogens exiting the body, they are trapped and move transversely back into the body. Interestingly, this is very often seen in conventional medicine. Although lesions are still discharging, patients are prescribed creams. The skin cannot breathe, the secretion or pus is trapped, and the healing process is thus impeded. The feedback of almost all patients is that they intuitively do not feel comfortable with creams when the wound still weeps.

Pastes (*Hú Jì* 糊剂)

Pastes are prepared by combining finely powdered herbs with a carrier substance. One type of paste is prepared using a greasy vehicle such as oil. In Chinese dermatology, sesame oil is very frequently used. The other type of paste is prepared with water. The paste is then rubbed on the affected area of the skin in order to protect dry skin, serve as a barrier, protect the affected area from bacterial infection, and promote the healing process of the skin.

Pastes should not be applied topically if there is profuse discharge. They should also be avoided in case of damp-heat (*shī rè* 湿热), as damp-heat could move transversely and the pathogenic process would be aggravated. Zōu Yuè pointed out in his *Wài Kē Zhēn Quán* (Personal Experience in Wài Kē, 1838) that "pastes are contraindicated when damp-heat toxins exist on the lower extremities. If misused, the confined heat will move transversely and spread even more extensively. Pastes are advisable in protected cases." Therefore, the application of pastes when the patient shows profuse pus or discharge will impede the drainage of the fluids.[14]

A very commonly used paste is *Jīn Huáng Sǎn* (Golden Yellow Powder)[15] mixed with an oil base. This paste is applied to a wide range of disorders in dermatology and trauma. It clears heat, resolves toxins, dispels dampness, eliminates blood stasis, and reduces swelling. It is thus very useful for inflammation, swellings, and pain in skin conditions such as carbuncles, acne, and insect bites.

Ointments (*Yóu Gāo* 油膏)

An ointment, also called a salve or balm, is a semi-solid preparation for external application on damaged skin. Oil-based ointments consist of finely powdered herbs heated in an oil base, such as almond oil, jojoba oil, or sesame oil. Sesame seeds are known to have the highest oil content. Sesame oil can be extracted from normal seeds or seeds that have been roasted prior to being processed. The oil of roasted sesame seeds is dark and smoky red, and has a distinctive aroma produced from the toasting and crushing of the seeds. This toasted sesame oil, often used in Chinese cooking, is particularly suitable for making oil-based ointments because it is comparatively stable and does not turn rancid on contact with air due to the toasting process. The texture of an oil-based ointment is thick and often looks yellowish. Creams, by contrast, are water-soluble and usually have a white hue. An ointment can be smoothly applied on damaged skin and it is absorbed easily and quickly.

Ointments usually have good permeability, and so they are often used after herbal baths and washes.

Oil-based ointments are often used to stop itching, clear heat, and dispel inflammation. Ointments are particularly suitable for chronic skin diseases or when the skin is very thick, such as seen in neurodermatitis. In psoriasis, the use of overly stimulating or irritating medicinals is contraindicated. If a patient has a very thick and scaly scalp, *Liú Huáng Gāo* (Sulfur Ointment) or *Huáng Lián Gāo* (Coptidis Balm)[16] are recommended. Ointments, like pastes, are contraindicated if there is profuse discharge.

Cream (*Rǔ Gāo* 乳膏)

A cream is a semi-solid emulsion of either oil-in-water or water-in-oil for topical use. Creams are spreadable substances, similar to ointments but not as thick, and they seem to be more appropriate for application on exposed skin areas such as the face and hands.

For compound creams, either oil-based herbal extracts or water-based herbal extracts (decoctions) are carefully blended with the base cream and other substances such as essential oils, aloe vera, or dexpanthenol[17] to achieve a homogenous and consistent product. In Chinese dermatology, base creams often consist of high-quality and skin-friendly substances such as shea butter, cocoa butter, jojoba oil, or natural white beeswax. It should be emphasized that Vaseline should not be used, although it is still often mentioned in medical textbooks. Vaseline, as a petroleum by-product of the oil industry, is not a high-quality solution. It is thick and often poorly spreadable. Cheap and low-quality substances such as Vaseline, paraffin, or propylene glycol usually leave a greasy film on the skin with increased sweating underneath. In sweating, salt crystals are produced, which would further worsen already existing itching, and therefore these substances should be avoided. For those who still prefer the use of Vaseline, wool wax alcoholic cream[18] can be used as an alternative. Wool wax alcoholic cream is a cream base, consisting of white Vaseline, cetyl-stearyl alcohol, and wool wax alcohol. Due to its lighter texture, it spreads easily and feels more pleasant on the skin.

However, when making your own creams and ointments, it is important to know exactly what ingredients are being used. Only pure, natural, environmentally friendly options should be used, ensuring that the ingredients do not irritate the skin and are suitable for sensitive skin care. Furthermore, if there is an ingredient a patient is allergic to, one can simply leave it out or replace it with something else.

Besides psoriasis, one instance in daily practice in which creams are frequently used is neurodermatitis. In neurodermatitis, lichenification can be seen; the skin is usually very dry, with scaling and itching. The patient feels very uncomfortable: as well as the visual effect and the itching sensation, the skin feels very tense. This is often quite painful. In this case creams made from herbs such as *shēng dì huáng, dāng guī, gān cǎo, sāng shèn*, or *bǎi hé* are frequently prescribed. It should be mentioned, however, that these kinds of creams should be only prescribed when the skin has healed and skin fissures are closed.

In order to treat the root cause of the disease, internal TCM remedies must be at the center of treatment. Nonetheless, external applications are often prescribed in addition. According to clinical experience, external treatments supplement and enhance the healing process, and the effect for the patient is more immediate. And we cannot underestimate the psychological factor here. The patient is more directly involved in the application of external remedies and thus can participate actively. This can be very important for some patients.

In the treatment of psoriasis, it should be pointed out that "soft" medicine needs to be used in any external treatment of psoriasis. This means non-irritating and low-concentrated medicinals with little or no perfume and additives in lotions and creams. Mildly composed compounds tend to work better as they are not too irritating and not too drying. Moreover, patients themselves are quite often very sensitive and easily have an allergic reaction to various kinds of external influences. Some patients say that they are even sensitive to water. This is why it is always advisable to take a mild approach instead of a harsh one when it comes to external treatments. However, just as with internal treatment, only an assessment of how the psoriasis lesions present can determine the best composition of any external application.

Endnotes

1 For example: Bensky, D., Clavey, S., and Stöger, E. (2004) *Materia Medica* (3rd edition). Seattle, WA: Eastland Press; or Chen, J.K. (2013) *Chinese Medical Herbology and Pharmacology*. City of Industry, CA: Art of Medicine Press.

2 Sòng Dynasty: Běi Sòng, Nán Sòng (Northern Sòng, Southern Sòng) (960–1279 AD).

3 Yuán Dynasty (1206–1368 AD).

4 Míng Dynasty (1368–1644 AD).

5 That is, TCM dermatologists.

6 Grant, J. (2003) *A Chinese Physician: Wang Ji and the Stone Mountain Medical Case Histories*. Abingdon: Routledge.

7 Qīng Dynasty (Before the Opium Wars of 1840) (1644–1911 AD).

8 With a pair of copper wires and a loop at the end of each wire.

9   Luo, H., Li, Q., Flower, A., Lewith, G., and Liu, J. (2012) "Comparison of effectiveness and safety between granules and decoction of Chinese herbal medicine: A systematic review of randomized clinical trials." *Journal of Ethnopharmacology 140,* 3, 555–567.

10   Sturgeon, S. (2012) *Powders and Granules RCHM.* Norwich: Register of Chinese Herbal Medicine.

11   Sturgeon, S. (2011) "Questions and answers about extract powders/granules–part one." *The Mayway Mailer,* November 2011. Accessed on 8/24/2019 at www.mayway.com/pdfs/maywaymailers/Skye-Sturgeon-QM-Extract-powder-11-2011.pdf.

12   Wu, Q., Christensen, LA., Legerski, R.J., and Vasquez, K.M. (2005) "Mismatch repair participates in error-free processing of DNA interstrand crosslinks in human cells." *EMBO Reports 6,* 6, 551–557.

13   Momtaz, K. and Fitzpatrick, T.B. (1998) "The benefits and risks of long-term PUVA photochemotherapy." *Dermatologic Clinics 16,* 2, 227–234

14   Taken from my TCM Dermatology seminar notes.

15   *Jīn Huáng Sǎn: huáng bǎi, dà huáng, jiāng huáng, bái zhǐ, hòu pò, chén pí, cāng zhú, tiān nán xīng, gān cǎo.*

16   Can be found in Appendix I.

17   Dexpanthenol, also known as panthenol, pantothenol, or provitamin B5, is often used as a moisturizer and to improve wound healing in creams, ointments, and lotions.

18   Wool wax or wool grease, also called lanolin.

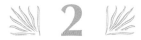

2

The Skin

ACCORDING TO TCM, the skin has a yáng character because it is located on the surface (outside) and is controlled by the Lungs. The skin is the main seat of the *wèi qì*, the defense qì, which warms, strengthens, and nourishes the skin. It also controls the opening and closing of the pores. A healthy skin is thus linked to an intact defense qì, and if these tasks are performed properly, our skin is healthy and resilient. The complexion looks bright and there are no pathological changes.

The Anatomical Structure of the Skin

The skin is our body's largest organ with a surface area of 1.5–2.0 m², and it is the one organ every person sees daily. This is certainly one of the reasons why patients are often quite depressed when they experience changes on their skin—because these changes are visible to themselves and everyone else. Many patients feel uncomfortable and ashamed, especially if the affected skin areas are located on the face or on the hands. Patients cover lesions up with make-up or clothes, but although that might help visually to some extent, it certainly is a great inconvenience and does not treat the problem itself.

The skin is the body's primary barrier against microbial pathogens, and it represents a unique environment in which immune cells interact with skin cells to maintain tissue homeostasis and induce immune responses. The skin has three layers: the epidermis, the dermis, and the subcutaneous fatty region. Each layer performs specific tasks, which will be described below. We should be aware that not all germs are bad. Commensal microbes, like bacteria, viruses, and fungi living on the skin, have beneficial effects in the protection against pathogens and facilitate wound healing. In a healthy balance, they form a perfect symbiosis to protect us. It is their imbalance that—as is commonly the case with imbalances—is harmful.

Epidermis

The epidermis, relatively thin and tough, acts as a shield for the body. It is an external elastic layer that is continuously regenerated every 28–30 days. The epidermis is composed of highly specialized epithelial cells, known as keratinocytes, which are arranged in multiple layers. They are continuously replenished from just one layer of basal keratinocytes that divide frequently. Dead skin cells called corneocytes form the upmost layer, which is largely responsible for the skin's barrier function. Scattered throughout the basal layer of the epidermis are cells called melanocytes. They synthesize the pigment melanin that protects against UV radiation and gives our skin its color.

Other epidermal cells are Langerhans cells, the antigen-presenting immune cells of the skin, and Merkel cells, the neuroendocrine cells functioning as mechanoreceptors. Langerhans cells directly interact with skin-resident memory T cells. They induce the activation and proliferation of skin-resident regulatory T cells, and they induce and control the proliferation of skin-resident effector memory T cells. These cells play a major role in the body's immune defense system. Merkel cells are deemed to be secondary sensory cells, as they are sensitive to touch and pressure. In case of an adequate irritant, they provoke an afferent excitation. Merkel cells are mainly found in sensitive skin regions, such as the fingertips and tip of the nose.

Dermis

The dermis is the layer beneath the epidermis. In the dermis, cells known as fibroblasts secrete elastin and collagen fibers that form a dense extracellular matrix. This extracellular matrix gives the skin its flexibility and strength. The dermis contains nerve endings, sweat glands and sebaceous glands, hair follicles, blood and lymph vessels, as well as mast cells. Blood vessels nourish the dermis, while lymph fluid is drained through the lymph vessels to the lymph nodes. Blood vessels also help regulate the temperature by dilating or contracting, which is why the skin pales when a person feels cold and reddens when he or she flushes.

Subcutis (Hypodermis)

Below the dermis lies the subcutaneous tissue, a layer of fat that helps insulate the body from heat and cold, provides protective padding for shock absorption, and allows the storage of fat for energy reserves. The fat remains in adipose (fat) cells, held together by fibrous tissue. It is surrounded by connective tissue, larger blood vessels, and nerves. The fatty layer varies in thickness, from very thin on the eyelids to several centimeters on the abdomen and gluteal region in some people.

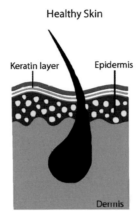

THE ANATOMY OF THE SKIN[1]

The Physiological Functions of the Skin

The skin performs a number of important functions. As the interface between the body and the environment, it plays a key role in protecting the body against external pathogens and forms a barrier for the exchange of fluids. Other functions are temperature control, sensation, and communication.

Protection

Due to the keratinization of the epithelium and glandular secretion, the skin forms an anatomical barrier to pathogens and damage. The skin serves as the body's defense system to the external environment. It protects the body against mechanical, chemical, and thermic damages. It also protects the body against the invasion of external microorganisms.

Immune Response

The skin is a dynamic organ and also participates in the body's immune-biological defense processes. It contains different cells, which are activated when the tissue is under attack by invading pathogens, such as the Langerhans cells, which are part of the adaptive (acquired) immune system.

Memory T cells patrol the skin and are capable of responding to repeated attackers from the outside, monocytes and mast cells. Memory T cells are T cells that have learned how to fight off an invader by "remembering" the strategy used to defeat previous infections. This mechanism is particularly important in gaining life-long immunity to infections such as scarlet fever, rubella, mumps, or chickenpox.

Temperature Control

Temperature control is the process of keeping the body at a constant temperature of 37°C. Sweat regulation and skin blood flow are both essential for maintaining the body's core temperature. Sweating begins almost precisely at a skin temperature of 37°C and increases rapidly as the skin temperature rises above this value, regulated by neural feedback mechanisms which operate primarily through the hypothalamus.[2] If skin temperature drops below 37°C, a variety of responses are initiated to preserve the heat within the body and to increase heat production. These include vasoconstriction to decrease the flow of heat to the skin, and cessation of sweating.

Water Resistance

The skin also acts as a barrier to water. Skin barrier function depends on the lipid-enriched stratum corneum cell membrane in the epidermis. Water resistance is important because it prevents the body from losing necessary nutrients and minerals.

Sensation

Another important function of the skin is detecting the different sensations of heat, cold, touch, pressure, vibration, tissue injury, and pain. Sensation is felt through a rich network of nerve endings with a variety of sensory receptors in the dermis.

Synthesis of Vitamin D

Vitamin D is crucial for building and maintaining strong bones. The synthesis of vitamin D is induced by UV light and is then transmuted in the Liver and in the Kidneys into a hormone called calcitriol. Calcitriol increases the blood calcium level by promoting the absorption of dietary calcium from the gastrointestinal tract into the blood. Calcitriol also stimulates the release of calcium from the bones. It thus affects the human bone's mineral density and bone turnover. Vitamin D deficiency causes osteomalacia, called rickets when it occurs in children.

Absorption and Excretion

Although the skin is a waterproof barrier, some substances such as certain drugs and remedies can be administered through the skin by means of ointments or adhesive patches and essential oils. Those substances can penetrate the skin through the layers, the hair follicles, and sweat glands. The concentration of penetration is limited by the skin's health and condition.

The skin serves as an excretory organ, disposing of waste material and toxins. Waste substances are expelled from the body through the skin via the sweat glands and normally take the form of salts, carbon dioxide, urea, and ammonia.

Not only is the skin our largest organ but it also carries great responsibility for our well-being. It protects us every single day. This is why it is so important to treat it well. A big problem is excessive personal hygiene, such as showering too often or with water that is too hot, using masses of shower gel, or, even worse, shower gel which contains chemicals, irritating substances, and perfume. Visits to the solarium and using chemicals are certainly not a good way to take care of our skin. These habits harm our skin, as it is no longer able to sustain its natural function as a barrier: the skin becomes irritated, dries out, and can no longer be nourished. Patients often need to reconsider their skin routines, and we need to create awareness for the importance of this organ, the skin, and how sensitive it is.

Endnotes

1 Illustration by Sabine Schmitz © 2018.

2 The hypothalamus is an important "control center" of our body. It is an area of the brain called the interbrain (diencephalon) and it is located below (= hypo) the thalamus. The hypothalamus contains not only control mechanisms for water, salt balance, and blood pressure, for instance, but also the key temperature sensors. It is also an important inceptor within the endocrine system because it regulates when and at what amount a hormone is formed.

3

The Western View
of Psoriasis

The Etiology and Definition of Psoriasis
According to Western Medicine

Psoriasis is a common systemic skin disease. It is characterized by chronic inflammation of the skin with changes in the maturation of keratinocytes, which manifests as dry, thickened, and silver-scaled plaques. According to our clinical observation, up to 50% of psoriasis cases start on the scalp (head). After several months or even many years, the lesions can spread all over the body. The lesions can also affect the trunk and the limbs at a later stage if no treatment occurs. In very mild cases, patients may not seek medical care. Reasons for this turn out to be that either the disease itself is not recognized as such or that the potential severity of the disease and its effects are underestimated. Therefore, when patients finally seek treatment, the exact moment when the psoriasis began is often difficult to determine.

Current research links psoriasis to an inflammatory and immune mechanism most likely associated with a genetic predisposition, but this has not yet been entirely confirmed. Psoriasis is associated with cardiovascular disease, depression, and psoriatic arthritis.[1] It is a burdensome disease, often causes considerable psychosocial disorders, and has a major impact on the patient's quality of life.[2]

Special attention should be paid to diagnosing psoriasis correctly in its early stages, because this condition is often misdiagnosed as dandruff if it starts on the scalp, or as other skin conditions such as seborrheic dermatitis or eczema. If initially misdiagnosed, it becomes difficult to treat and takes longer to respond. It is amazing how many patients have experienced exactly this process: a long-standing pathogenesis and the disease itself either not recognized as a skin disorder or misdiagnosed, and therefore mistreated.

This often means that patients we see in our practices have a very long medical history and have often already received various conventional medical therapies.

Prevalence of Psoriasis Worldwide

Psoriasis is very often seen in clinics, and the course and progress of psoriasis is often unpredictable due to environmental factors, lifestyle habits, and, as stated above, reaching the correct diagnosis in time and subsequently receiving proper treatment. To expand our perspective, it is interesting to provide a larger context by looking at trends in the incidence of psoriasis worldwide.

Psoriasis is prevalent worldwide, but its frequency varies in relation to demographic characteristics, race, and geographic region. Its global prevalence is relatively high and consistently quoted at around 2%.[3] In the different populations it ranges from 0% (Samoa) to 11.8% (Arctic-Kasach'ye).[4] The data available on individual regions worldwide show that the prevalence in adults aged 20 and older is 3.2% in the United States.[5] In Europe the estimated prevalence varies from 0.6 to 6.5%.[6] In Norway, for example, it exceeds this figure at 8.5%.[7] Population-based surveys from China and Japan have given prevalence ranging from 0.05 to 1.23% and 0.29 to 1.18%. Similar rates were found in India with 0.5 to 2.3%.[8]

The foregoing data concern adults. With regard to children, we can state that although psoriasis can occur at any age, it is less common in children than in adults, as the following data show. In general, the prevalence of psoriasis in children is up to 0.71% in Europe.[9] In Italy, for example, a lifetime prevalence of psoriasis of 2.15%[10] was found, diagnosed by a dermatologist. In Germany, a study based on an insurance database and confined to minors under 18 years reported an overall prevalence of psoriasis in children of 0.71% and the prevalence seems to increase with age.[11] Interestingly, psoriasis in children is almost absent in Asia.[12] Data show that psoriasis can develop at any age, but in about 75% of patients with psoriasis the onset is before the age of 40 years. Only in about 25% of patients does it appear before the age of 20 years.[13]

As mentioned above, the global prevalence of psoriasis also seems to vary in relation to ethnic groups. So far, epidemiological data of psoriasis in relation to race are rare and there is no definite explanation for these variations in frequency. Although the data in non-Caucasian populations are limited, it suggests that psoriasis is more common in white people. Studies found that the prevalence of psoriasis at all ages is overall lower in non-Caucasian populations, with zero cases in the Indian population of Latin America, 0.19% in Egypt, 0.44% in Sri Lanka, 0.23% in Taiwan, and 0.123–0.35% in China.[14] Available data from the United States report the highest prevalence in Caucasians at 3.6%, followed by African Americans at 1.9% and Hispanics at 1.6%.[15] Moreover, studies in Australia found a prevalence of 2.6% in Caucasians and no cases in the Aboriginal population.[16]

There are also differences between geographic regions and the occurrence of psoriasis. Worldwide, the variation in the prevalence of psoriasis appears to depend on the distance from the equator, with populations located closer to the equator such as Egypt, Tanzania, Sri Lanka, and Taiwan being less affected by psoriasis compared with countries and continents more distant from it, such as Europe and Australia.[17] A valid question therefore is if this might be caused by the differences in exposure to the UV wavelength of sunlight. Psoriasis often gets better in summer and worse in winter, so sunlight definitely has a protective role. The more UV radiation the body gets, the smaller the chance that the disease will spread. This might explain the low frequency of psoriasis in certain African countries. On the other hand, this cannot explain the difference between black and non-black Americans in the United States. It has not been confirmed beyond doubt, but there might be some genetic factors promoting resistance to psoriasis in certain groups of the human population, plus environmental influences such as weather, cultural habits, and socioeconomic factors which could explain these observed differences.[18]

This larger context leads directly to the most common risk factors of psoriasis. Factors such as dietary habits as well as the consumption of tobacco and alcohol obviously play an important role in the differences between geographic regions and races worldwide. Fatty food and high tobacco and alcohol consumption are quite clearly more common in the so-called "Western lifestyle" and Western countries. In any of the Asian countries, where the incidence of psoriasis is reported as lower, this lifestyle is rather uncommon. However, we might assume that lifestyle and dietary habits in the Asian countries will change over time—for instance, in China where living standards are rising and lifestyle habits are being adapted to the West. A classic example is the consumption of fast food.

The fact that the worldwide prevalence of psoriasis is around 2% (studies in developed countries have reported prevalence rates of on average 4.6%)[19] makes psoriasis a serious inflammatory skin disease, which is worthy of being addressed in detail in order to find new treatment solutions for literally millions of patients.

Risk Factors According to Western Medicine

Trends in the occurrence of psoriasis show a significant increase over time.[20] During the last three decades the annual incidence almost doubled.[21] The rise can certainly not be explained by known genetic factors alone. There are many factors to be considered, but obvious reasons include environmental changes or environmental influences, lifestyle changes, and increased stress or psycho-emotional aspects caused by changes in society. The numbers could also simply reflect changes in diagnosing patterns over time. Compared with three decades ago, for example, the standard and precision in medical diagnosing techniques and medical care has improved enormously.

What has been confirmed so far is that psoriasis can be triggered by interactions between multiple genetic factors and different environmental factors[22] or infections including the common cold, upper respiratory infections, tonsillitis, and streptococcal throat infections such as pharyngitis. Streptococcal infection is most commonly associated with a group A beta-hemolytic streptococcus infection, which is a gram-positive bacterium and responsible for a wide range of infections. Psoriasis itself is not contagious. In the clinic it can be very often observed that psychological stress can influence the course of the disease.[23] It is not uncommon for patients to report that their skin has got worse after some excitement, following an argument, or during work overload. Often, exacerbations can be seen relatively soon or a few days after a stressful event. Concerning genetic factors, a family history of psoriasis cannot be ignored, as there is a strong association between psoriasis and a family history of psoriasis.[24] But genes cover just one aspect of possible triggering factors.

A number of other risk factors are recognized which can worsen the disease, such as certain foods, alcohol, smoking,[25] obesity, abrupt discontinuation of systemic superpotent topical corticosteroids,[26] antihypertensive drugs, and herbal patent formulas for joint pain. Chinese herbal patent formulas often contain warming herbs. If we consider that psoriasis is an inflammatory disease, heat is always involved at a progressed stage. Thus, warming herbs are contraindicated. Factors such as the seasons also need to be considered. As mentioned previously, psoriasis often worsens in winter. Finally, patients with HIV infection and an acquired immune deficiency may also be more vulnerable to an exacerbation of psoriasis.[27]

Different Types of Psoriasis Manifestation

Psoriasis can present as various types: genotype psoriasis, sub-clinical (geno-phenotypical) psoriasis, and phenotypical (clinically manifest) psoriasis.

Genotype Psoriasis

As mentioned above, a significant risk factor for developing psoriasis is having a family history of the disease, particularly if the patient's parents suffer from it. However, in genotype psoriasis, the patient has a corresponding predisposition without presenting any manifestation of the disease. In the clinic this means we need to consider that a genetic factor, which has been not accurately identified, makes an outbreak of psoriasis possible. The genetic factor determines the genotype of a likely development of psoriasis. In order to stimulate the actual outbreak of the disease, the transition from genotype to phenotype and the externally visible skin disease, there need to be triggering factors. Psoriasis can, but does not have to, erupt. The number of patients carrying genotype psoriasis is not definitively known because no exact data have been gathered. Without an outbreak of the disease, all data are just speculative.

Sub-clinical or Geno-phenotypical Psoriasis

The sub-clinical or geno-phenotypical type of psoriasis is a clinical mix between genotype and phenotype psoriasis. The patient has minimal skin changes such as silvery white dandruff, low scaling on the elbow and knees, implied psoriatic nail changes, and redness and scaling in different skin areas. Small lesions, and lesions located in concealed areas, are quite often overlooked and not identified as psoriasis. In those patients it is quite helpful to ask about a family history of psoriasis.

Phenotypical or Clinically Manifest Psoriasis

In the phenotypical or clinically manifest type, psoriasis can be observed in its complete severity and it is further divided into different subcategories, which we will come back to later.

Psoriasis in its classical form is easy to diagnose. In contrast, the sub-clinical forms are more difficult to diagnose correctly. To reach the right diagnosis, particularly in atypical variations, an examination of the entire skin is the only option. Moreover, to ensure that mild forms with only individual lesions are not missed, if psoriasis is indicated, the following body parts should be examined in detail: behind the ear, the navel, the anal folds, and the scalp.

The Mechanism of Psoriasis According to Conventional Medicine

In order to fully understand the benefits of TCM treatment, it is useful to discuss the current perspective of conventional medicine and its shortcomings. The symptom-related treatment that conventional medicine offers in no way treats the cause of disease. Even if the root cause is taken into consideration, which is almost never the case, it does not offer satisfactory explanations for what causes the disease. It may therefore not be possible for conventional medicine to give a cause-related treatment, and thus its long-term effectiveness must be questioned.

Despite great progress in research, the primary cause of psoriasis has still not been determined. So far it has become clear that it is an inheritable disease, but the exact inheritance mode remains unclear.[28] When discussing possible pathogenetic factors, two important characteristics of psoriatic tissue reactions are at the foreground: inflammation and massive epidermal hyperproliferation. This means that psoriasis is mainly characterized by excessively increased keratinocyte proliferation, accelerated angiogenesis, vasodilation, and in situ detection of autoreactive T cells. Several lines of evidence support the idea that psoriasis appears to depend on T cells infiltrating skin lesions, which, it has been proposed, mediate the disease through an autoimmune process. Certainly, autoimmunity does not appear to be the only component in the development of psoriasis. Psoriasis is, however, a manifestation of several skin immune reactions, but inflammation is the limiting key feature of the pathogenesis in this disease. For a better understanding of the complex pathophysiology of psoriasis, it is important to know exactly what happens in the skin.

A Complex Chessboard: The Immunopathogenesis of Psoriasis

Psoriasis is, as explained above, characterized by changes in the maturation of keratinocytes, which manifest in a hyperproliferation of the epidermis. The formation rate of the cells significantly increases so that the epidermis is thicker than in its normal state. Those cells, formed in large quantities, do not have enough time for maturation and reach the surface of the skin within a few days only. It has been demonstrated that the keratinocytes of psoriatic patients have a significant shortening of their cell cycle from about 311 hours in normal persons to only 36 hours,[29] and the turnover time of the epidermis is distinctly shortened from 26–27 days to four days.[30] This results in a massive accumulation of immature skin cells that become visible as silvery scales seen in sharply defined, scaly reddish plaques at the surfaces of the skin. The question remains, though, as to what provokes this change in the maturation of keratinocytes.

Immunological research has accumulated evidence on an alteration of the innate immune system (keratinocytes, neutrophils, mast cells, endothelial cells, dendritic cells) and the adaptive immune system, particularly T cells, in patients with psoriasis. A deeper look at the whole process will be helpful in understanding this further. A psoriatic plaque is induced and maintained by multiple interactions between cells of the skin and a dysregulated immune system. It seems to be an epidermal problem of faulty epidermopoesis (epidermal turnover) due to impaired autocontrol mechanisms, mediated by T lymphocyte immune cells and their secretory products, cytokines. These cytokines, such as transforming growth factor (TGF) and vascular endothelial growth factor (VEGF)–both inducing angiogenesis–are activated and will lead to an excessive proliferation of keratinocytes, epidermal hyperplasia, angiogenesis, and significant vasodilation. VEGF over-expression in the skin lesions accelerates angiogenesis and increases vascular permeability, which is caused by the migration of inflammatory cells. As VEGF promotes the division and proliferation of endothelial cells, it is thought to promote the pathological process of psoriasis. VEGF levels in lesion tissue are much higher than in normal skin. The immune-regulatory cells play an important role in the maintenance of normal immune balance. The balance between regulatory T cells and effector T cells is extremely important for a normal process. Regulatory T cells inhibit the independent activation of T cells and maintain self-tolerance.[31] In psoriasis, this self-regulation no longer exists. In this scenario, psoriasis is similar to other inflammatory diseases of the bowel such as colitis, or of the joints such as rheumatoid arthritis. The cluster of symptoms of all those inflammatory diseases is inconsistent but surely has a basic, pathogenetic path mediated by T cells, with a polygenic inheritance probably due to several genetic defects.

Another important aspect is the swelling of the skin in psoriasis that very often occurs. This is because the dermis contains a large number of blood and lymph vessels as well as nerve endings. The affected area of the skin reddens with the dilatation of small blood vessels and increased blood supply due to the inflammatory response. An increased number of immune cells and fluid enter into the tissue, which results in an accumulation of fluids in the affected area and leads to swelling of the skin.

A further typical finding of psoriasis is the so-called "Auspitz phenomenon"[32] (in TCM it is called *xuè lù xiàn xiàng* 血露现象), in which the removal of a scale leads to pinpoint bleeding, usually after scratching. This happens because the epidermal layer overlying the tips of the dermal papillae is thinning out, and blood vessels within the papillae are dilated and tortuous, and bleed readily when the scale is removed.[33] This phenomenon is also called "bloody dew" and it is a clear diagnostic sign of psoriasis vulgaris.

Looking at the immunopathogenesis of psoriasis as described above, it can be said that the entire process is a vicious cycle of proliferation and inflammation of the skin, characterized by hyperproliferation of keratinocytes in the epidermis. Unfortunately, conventional medicine has so far been unable to determine a sustainable treatment for psoriasis.

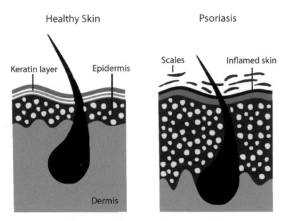

HEALTHY SKIN VS. PSORIASIS[34]

Current Treatment Options in Western Medicine

The concept of conventional therapy for psoriasis until now has been derived from its immunopathogenesis—that is, from integrating knowledge about interactions between the cells of the immune system and their cytokines, which initiate pathologic processes and finally lead to a development of the typical clinical features of psoriasis: inflammation and hyperproliferation of the epidermis.

Consequently, these mechanisms seem of enormous significance in the treatment of psoriasis: controlling the immune and inflammatory response by directly targeting the inflammatory cascade and blocking specific cytokines such as TGF or VEGF. Even though all this is known, a cure for the disease has not been found. As psoriasis is a chronic relapsing disease, it may require a very long period of treatment. Treatment modalities are local therapy and/or systemic therapy, and can also be found in the form of phototherapy, which can be combined with other forms of therapy.

Systemic Treatments
Acitretin

Acitretin is known to be a systemic treatment and it is used to treat severe and very severe forms of common psoriasis (psoriasis vulgaris). Acitretin belongs to the group of retinoids (vitamin A acid derivatives), known to have anti-proliferative and immune-modulating properties. Used in treating skin diseases, acitretin influences the mitotic activity and differentiation of keratinocytes. It slows the intra-epidermal migration of neutrophilic granulocytes and inhibits interleukin-6 (IL-6)-induced development of T helper cells (TH17 cells), which play an important role in the pathogenesis of psoriasis and the differentiation of regulatory T cells.[35] Retinoids such as acitretin intervene in this system to regulate the uncontrolled growth of skin cells and promote the slow maturation of the newly formed cells.

Although the symptoms of psoriasis can be alleviated by this therapy, there can be no change to the root cause of the disease. The list of common side effects of acitretin is long. These include back pain, joint pain, a ringing or buzzing or other unexplained noise in the ears, excessive muscle tension, headache, muscle stiffness, and insomnia.[36] The possible side effects of this treatment might be even more unpleasant than the psoriasis itself.

Cyclosporine

Cyclosporine is also subcategorized as a systemic treatment. It is an immunosuppressive drug, which suppresses the immune system and slows down the growth of certain immune cells. An important mechanism in the activation of T cells is the nuclear translocation of factors that can increase the expression of pro-inflammatory mediators. Through its inhibitory effect on the production of important immunological mediators, especially in T cells, it is considered to be a selective immunosuppressant. Its effect is reversible and it has no myelotoxic or mutagenic properties.[37]

Besides the desired effects, cyclosporine may cause many unwanted side effects.[38] Cyclosporine, as an immunosuppressant, may leave patients vulnerable to infections. It can cause high blood pressure and kidney problems. Moreover, psoriasis patients who have had previous treatments with cyclosporine have an increased risk of developing skin cancer. Therefore, the benefit must be carefully weighed against potential risks. As with acitretin, cyclosporine must be given only under close medical supervision.

Methotrexate

Methotrexate (MTX) is given as a systemic treatment and was initially used to treat cancer. It has anti-inflammatory effects and regulates the misdirected immune system (immune-modulatory effects). MTX engages cellular metabolism. In psoriasis, MTX inhibits an enzyme involved in the rapid growth of skin cells and slows down their growth rate. As MTX is a drug that heavily intervenes with the immunological processes of the human organism, it needs very regular medical supervision. It has, like other cytotoxic substances, a broad array of possible side effects[39] including nausea, vomiting, diarrhea, dizziness, and stomach and joint pain. Delayed side effects such as bone marrow suppression may also be possible.

Topical Treatments
Steroids (Corticosteroids)

Steroids are the most commonly prescribed drugs for topical treatment of mild to moderate cases of psoriasis. Steroids, such as prednisone or deltasone, work by reducing inflammation and slowing down the growth and build-up of skin cells. If they are used too frequently, patients may develop serious skin damage, such as skin thinning, changes in pigmentation, easy bruising, stretch marks, redness, and dilated surface blood vessels. If steroids are taken over long periods of time, they can also affect internal organs,[40] because they can be absorbed through the skin. A further disadvantage is that they are not sustainable: the symptoms will reappear soon after drug cessation.

The types of corticosteroids and method of treatment are chosen depending on the location of the affected region. For the scalp and hairline, foams and shampoos are available. Ointments are more suitable for thicker skin lesions such as the skin on elbows and knees, whereas creams are suitable for thinner skin lesions. It should be mentioned that this type of treatment is very time-consuming, as patients have to apply it every day. This may result in lower patient compliance, and since this form of treatment depends on regularity, lack of compliance means reduced efficacy.

Vitamin D3 Derivatives

Well-known vitamin D3 derivatives such as calcitriol, tacalcitol, and calcipotriol are available as the current first-line intervention for psoriasis vulgaris. They can be used as monotherapy but are often combined with topical corticosteroids in ointments or creams. The biologically active forms of calcitriol, tacalcitol, and calcipotriol are known to normalize cell differentiation, cell proliferation, and immunomodulation.[41] The treatment with calcitriol, for example, shows a relatively good tolerability. Side effects are usually not severe, although slight systemic effects on calcium levels and calcium secretion seem to characterize the safety profile.[42]

UV Phototherapy

Phototherapy (sunlight therapy) has long been used for the treatment of skin conditions. The use of modern ultraviolet (UV) phototherapy, specifically for the treatment of psoriasis, is a more recent development, starting in the early 20th century.[43] Compared with other therapy methods, UV phototherapy is relatively simple to apply: patients expose their skin to an artificial UV light source on a regular basis. This form of treatment can be done under medical supervision in clinics or at home, making it an economical and convenient choice for many patients.

In phototherapy, it is important to distinguish between broadband (UVA) and narrowband (UVB) light. The major difference between broadband and narrowband is that narrowband UVB light units release a more specific or smaller (narrow) range of ultraviolet light. Potential effects and related side effects also have to be taken into consideration. Recently, the application of broadband treatment has been discouraged and narrowband treatment is now preferred, as it seems to be more effective and causes fewer side effects.[44]

UVB Phototherapy

In UVB phototherapy, UVB light penetrates the skin and slows down the excessive growth of affected skin cells. The efficacy of this therapy can be increased by the application of topical remedies. For example, in combination with the application of "Dead Sea Salt" baths as a form of so-called balneotherapy, UVB has an anti-inflammatory effect. In addition, the immune system of the skin can be influenced by the sole action of UVB light. Unfortunately, after UVB exposure the skin may redden, itch, and burn. The skin may also worsen temporarily before improving.

UVA Phototherapy

UVA light[45] phototherapy is a therapy combining UVA radiation with psoralen, but this is very rarely used in clinics nowadays. Traditional broadband UVA treatment has been replaced almost completely by narrowband UVB treatment. Like UVB light, UVA light carries a cumulative risk of cutaneous malignancy.[46]

Advantages and Disadvantages of Current Treatment Options in Western Medicine

It seems quite clear that conventional therapy can alleviate the symptoms of psoriasis only for a short time, without any impact on the underlying cause of the disease (proved when the symptoms of the disease reoccur after drug cessation). All these treatments are predominantly symptom-focused. Moreover, most conventional drugs such as corticosteroids have severe side effects, and immunosuppressive drugs such as methotrexate and cyclosporine that are often used to treat psoriasis interfere with the immunological processes of the human organism and thus cause undesired reactions. Patients taking such drugs need regular medical supervision, and it is the prescribing doctor's responsibility to weigh the use of such drugs against their inherent risks in order to give patients the best possible treatment and quality of life. In addition, the costs to both patients and healthcare systems of conventional medical drugs are relatively high[47] and patients frequently aren't comfortable taking them.

There is often no alternative in Western medicine, and corticosteroids or immunosuppressive drugs are prescribed if there is an inflammatory process as in psoriasis. Unfortunately, patients are often insufficiently informed about possible results and side effects of these drugs; concerns are not taken seriously, and allopaths generally suffer from constant time constraints in clinic. The time factor, however, is essential in a successful treatment of skin diseases. Conversations, listening, gathering information, and dealing with concerns form a vital part of the treatment. All in all, a suitable form of therapy for psoriasis that is effective and without extensive side effects must be found. And TCM treatment can certainly offer this.

Endnotes

1 Griffiths, C.E.M. and Barker, J.N.W.N. (2007) "Pathogenesis and clinical features of psoriasis." *Lancet 370*, 9583, 263–271.

2 Rapp, S.R., Feldman, S.R., Exum, M.L., Fleischer, A.B., Jr, and Reboussin, D.M. (1999) "Psoriasis causes as much disability as other major medical diseases." *Journal of the American Academy of Dermatology 41*, 3, 401–407.

3 Christophers, E. (2001) "Psoriasis–epidemiology and clinical spectrum." *Clinical and Experimental Dermatology 26*, 4, 314–320.

4 Farber, E.M. and Nall, L. (1998) "Epidemiology: Natural History and Genetics." In H.H. Roenigk Jr and H.I. Maibach (eds) *Psoriasis*. New York, NY: Dekker.

5 Rachakonda, T.D., Schupp, C.W., and Armstrong, A.W. (2014) "Psoriasis prevalence among adults in the United States." *Journal of the American Academy of Dermatology 70*, 3, 512–516.

6 Chandran, V. and Raychaudhuri, S.P. (2010) "Geoepidemiology and environmental factors of psoriasis and psoriatic arthritis." *Journal of Autoimmunity 34*, 3, J314–J321.

7 Parisi, R., Symmons, D.P., Griffiths, C.E., and Ashcroft, D.M. (2013) "Global epidemiology of psoriasis: A systematic review of incidence and prevalence." *Journal of Investigative Dermatology 133*, 2, 377–385.

8 Diallo, M. (2012) "Psoriasis epidemiology." *Journal of Clinical Case Reports 2*, 8, e116.

9 Augustin, M., Glaeske, G., and Radtke, M.A. (2010) "Epidemiology and comorbidity of psoriasis in children." *British Journal of Dermatology 162*, 633–636.

10 Naldi, L., Parazzini, F., Gallus, S., and GISED Study Centres (2009) "Prevalence of atopic dermatitis in Italian schoolchildren: Factors affecting its variation." *Acta Dermato-Venereologica 89*, 2, 122–125.

11 Augustin, M., Glaeske, G., and Radtke, M.A. (2010) "Epidemiology and comorbidity of psoriasis in children." *British Journal of Dermatology 162*, 633–636.

12 Chen, G.Y., Cheng, Y.W., and Wang, C.Y. (2008) "Prevalence of skin diseases among schoolchildren in Magong, Penghu, Taiwan: A community-based clinical survey." *Journal of Formosan Medical Association 107*, 1, 21–29.

13 WHO, Executive Board, 133rd session, EB133/5, April 5, 2013.

14 Parisi, R., Symmons, D.P., Griffiths, C.E., and Ashcroft, D.M. (2013) "Global epidemiology of psoriasis: A systematic review of incidence and prevalence." *Journal of Investigative Dermatology 133*, 2, 377–385.

15 Rachakonda, T.D., Schupp, C.W., and Armstrong, A.W. (2014) "Psoriasis prevalence among adults in the United States." *Journal of the American Academy of Dermatology 70*, 3, 512–516.

16 Farber, E.M. and Nall, L. (1994) "Psoriasis in the tropics: Epidemiologic, genetic, clinical, and therapeutic aspects." *Dermatologic Clinics 12*, 4, 805–816.

17 Parisi, R., Symmons, D.P., Griffiths, C.E., and Ashcroft, D.M. (2013) "Global epidemiology of psoriasis: A systematic review of incidence and prevalence." *Journal of Investigative Dermatology 133*, 2, 377–385,

18 Diallo, M. (2012) "Psoriasis epidemiology." *Journal of Clinical Case Reports 2*, 8, e116.

19 Parisi, R., Symmons, D.P., Griffiths, C.E., and Ashcroft, D.M. (2013) "Global epidemiology of psoriasis: A systematic review of incidence and prevalence." *Journal of Investigative Dermatology 133*, 2, 377–385.

20 Huerta, C., Rivero, E., and Rodriguez, L.A. (2007) "Incidence and risk factors for psoriasis in the general population." *Archives of Dermatology 143*, 12, 1559–1565.

21 Icen, M., Crowson, C.S., McEvoy, M.T., Dann, F.J., Gabriel, S.E., and Maradit Kremers, H. (2009) "Trends in incidence of adult-onset psoriasis over three decades: A population-based study." *Journal of the American Academy of Dermatology 60*, 3, 394–401.

22 Bowcock, A.M. and Barker, J.N. (2003) "Genetics of psoriasis: The potential impact on new therapies." *Journal of the American Academy of Dermatology 49*, suppl. 2, S51–56.

23 Seville, R.H. (1977) "Psoriasis and stress." *British Journal of Dermatology* 97, 279–302.

24 Naldi, L., Peli, L., Parazzini, F., Carrel, C.F., and Psoriasis Study Group of the Italian Group of Epidemiological Research in Dermatology (2001) "Family history of psoriasis, stressful life events, and recent infectious disease are risk factors for a first episode of acute guttate psoriasis: Results of a case-control study." *Journal of the American Academy of Dermatology 44*, 3, 433–438.

25 Higgins, E. (2000) "Alcohol, smoking and psoriasis." *Clinical and Experimental Dermatology 25*, 2, 107–110.

26 Abel, E.A., DiCicco, L.M., Orenberg, E.K., Fraki, J.E., and Farber, E.M. (1986) "Drugs in exacerbation of psoriasis." *Journal of the American Academy of Dermatology 15*, 1007–1022.

27 Lazar, A.P. and Roenigk, H.H. (1988) "Acquired immunodeficiency syndrome (AIDS) can exacerbate psoriasis." *Journal of the American Academy of Dermatology 18*, 144.

28 Christophers, E. (2003) *Psoriasis* (2nd edition). Berlin: Blackwell Verlag.

29 Van Scott, E.J. and Ekel, T.M. (1963) "Kinetics of hyperplasia in psoriasis." *Archives of Dermatology 88*, 373–381.

30 Weinstein, G.D. and Frost, P. (1968) "Abnormal cell proliferation in psoriasis." *Journal of Investigative Dermatology 150*, 254–258.

31 Hong, L. and Hong, H.J. (2012) "Research progress in immunopathogenesis of psoriasis." *Pharmaceutical Care and Research 12*, 4, 277–279.

32 Diagnosed by the German dermatologist Heinrich Auspitz at the end of the 19th century.

33 Kumar, V.L., Abbas, A., Fausto, N., Aster, J., *et al.* (2010) *Robbin's Textbook of Pathology.* New Delhi: Elsevier, p.841.

34 Illustration by Sabine Schmitz © 2018.

35 Leitlinie zur Therapie der Psoriasis vulgaris Update 2011, AWMF-Register (awmf.org).

36 www.nlm.nih.gov/medlineplus/druginfo.

37 Leitlinie zur Therapie der Psoriasis vulgaris Update 2011, AWMF-Register (awmf.org).

38 US Food and Drug Administration (FDA), NEORAL data sheet (Novartis), revised September 2009.

39 US Food and Drug Administration (FDA), Methotrexate data sheet, Ref. 3033070, revised October 2011.

40 US Food and Drug Administration (FDA), RAYOS (prednisone) data sheet, Ref. 3165107, revised July 2012.

41 Ellis, C.N., Berberian, B., Sulica, V.I., Dodd, W.A., *et al.* (1993) "A double-blind evaluation of topical capsaicin in pruritic psoriasis." *Journal of the American Academy of Dermatology 29*, 3, 438–442.

42 Chiricozzi, A. and Chimenti, S. (2012) "Effective topical agents and emerging perspectives in the treatment of psoriasis." *Expert Review of Dermatology 7*, 3, 283–293.

43 Wong, T., Hsu, L., and Liao, W. (2013) "Phototherapy in psoriasis: A review of mechanisms of action." *Journal of Cutaneous Medicine 17*, 1, 6–12.

44 Zhao, M., Guo, J., and Jia, H. (1999) "Light quantum oxygen transmission on compound Salvia miltiorrhiza fluid for psoriasis vulgaris." *Ningxia Medical Journal 21*, 5, 310.

45 Also known as long-wave light.

46 MacDonald, A. and Burden, A.D. (2007) "Psoriasis: Advances in pathophysiology and management." *Postgraduate Medical Journal 83*, 985, 690–697.

47 Javitz, H.S., Ward, M.M., Farber, E., Nail, L., *et al.* (2002) "The direct cost of care for psoriasis and psoriatic arthritis in the United States." *Journal of the American Academy of Dermatology 46*, 850–860.

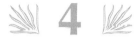

4

The TCM Perspective on Psoriasis

The Historical Naming of Psoriasis in Traditional Chinese Medicine

TCM now refers to psoriasis as *bái bǐ* 白疕 (white crust). This has not always been the case: psoriasis had had multiple other labels and names in ancient literature until TCM finally settled on this term.

Many ancient TCM books describe psoriasis. From ancient times to now, the Chinese have referred to psoriasis by many names: the aforementioned *bái bǐ* 白疕 (white crust), as well as *niú pí xuǎn* 牛皮癣 (pine skin tinea or alternatively cow skin eczema), *sōng pí xuǎn* 松皮癣 (a kind of ringworm), *gān xuǎn* 干癣 (dry ringworm), *fēng xuǎn* 风癣 (wind ringworm), *shé fēng* 蛇风 (snake wind), and *wán xuǎn* 顽癣 (prolonged ringworm). In addition to all these names, terms such as *bái ké chuāng* 白壳疮 (named by its silver scales) or *jīn qián fēng* 金钱风 (the size of its skin lesion is as big as copper and the color is silver) have appeared as well.

The colloquial name *niú pí xuǎn* originates from *Yī Zōng Jīn Jiàn* (The Golden Mirror of Ancestral Medicine, c. 1736–1743), written by Wú Qiān *et al.* The book describes six types of "*xuǎn*" (ringworm) and clearly distinguishes *sōng pí xuǎn* from *niú pí xuǎn*:

> The fourth "*xuǎn*" is called *niú pí xuǎn*. The skin lesion feels like the skin of an ox's neck, thick and firm. The fifth "*xuǎn*" is called *sōng pí xuǎn* and the skin lesion of this type feels like the coating of a pine tree, characterized by whitish lesions connected to reddish lesions and an itching sensation.[1]

However, at the present time psoriasis is mostly called *bái bǐ* (white crust), as it appears in dotted form with white marks.

The Definition and History of Psoriasis According to Traditional Chinese Medicine

Now that TCM has settled on a name for the disease, it is interesting to explore the history of psoriasis and how the perspective on it has changed (or been expanded) during the last 1500 years.

c. 1065–771 BC	*Wŭ Shí Èr Bìng Fāng* (Prescriptions for Fifty-Two Diseases), author unknown[2]	▪ Seemingly earliest reference to the term "*bĭ*" ▪ Records *shēn bĭ* 身疕 (*bĭ* over the trunk) ▪ Character *bĭ* 疕 at that time mainly meant external injuries
Suí Dynasty[3] 610 AD	*Zhū Bìng Yuán Hóu Lùn* (General Treatise on the Etiology and Symptomology of Diseases), by Cháo Yuánfāng	▪ Earliest ancient description of psoriasis from TCM perspective ▪ Description of a disease called *gān xiăn* (*xiăn* = lichen) ▪ Manifestation of the lesions: "The boundary of skin lesions is evident. … Epidermis is thickening, shriveled, cracking, and itching. … Silver scales will be drawing off when the epidermis is scratched"[4] ▪ Pathogenesis: pathogenic factors combine wind (*fēng* 风), dampness (*shī* 湿), and toxin (*dú* 毒), which invade the exterior skin
Táng Dynasty[5] 752 AD	*Wài Tái Mì Yào* (Arcane Essentials from the Imperial Library), by Wáng Tāo	▪ Mentions that the etiology of psoriasis is mainly due to wind and dampness in the skin combined with an imbalance between cold-dampness, qì, and blood ▪ At this time, a lot of external applications for psoriasis were first reported, which were mostly used for the elimination of dampness and parasites, e.g. worms
Early Míng Dynasty 1575	*Yī Xué Rù Mén* (Introduction to Medicine), by Lĭ Chān	▪ First time: psoriasis caused mainly by blood heat and wind dryness ▪ Leads to wind toxin that invades skin
Míng Dynasty 1602	*Zhèng Zhì Zhŭn Shéng* (Standard Differentiation of Patterns and Treatments), by Wáng Kĕntáng	▪ Psoriasis most likely caused by invasion of combined dampness and heat in Spleen (*pí* 脾) channel ▪ Also by external invasion of wind-heat in Lung (*fèi* 肺) ▪ Manifestation is generalized all over body with skin lesions eroding and diffuse ▪ Patient's skin itches and aches–course of disease prolonged ▪ *Bái bĭ* (white *bĭ*) is rather described as symptom
Míng Dynasty 1617	*Wài Kē Zhèng Zōng* (Compendium on External Diseases Traditional Chinese Medicine), by Chén Shígōng	▪ Cause is described as the combination of wind (*fēng xuăn*–wind ringworm), heat, dampness (*shī xuăn* 湿癣–dampness ringworm), and insects

Qīng Dynasty 1665	*Wài Kē Dà Chéng* (Great Compendium of External Medicine), by Qí Kūn	• *Bái bǐ* first described as a "name" of specific disease • "The skin lesion of the patient with *bái bǐ* is like that of measles and scabies, whitish and itching, with silver scales, also known as *shé fēng* (snake wind)"[6] • Pathogenic wind and blood dryness as cause, malnourishment of the skin as the result
Qīng Dynasty 1740	*Wài Kē Zhèng Zhì Quán Shēng Jí* (Compendium of Patterns and Treatments in External Medicine), by Wáng Wéi Dé	• Psoriasis mostly caused by autumn-dryness, blood deficiency, and a weak constitution • Scales emerge after scratching, developing to dried-up, chapped/cracked skin • Corresponding treatment methods of moisturizing dryness by nourishing the blood and activating blood circulation were advocated
Qīng Dynasty c. 1736–1743	*Yī Zōng Jīn Jiàn* (The Golden Mirror of Ancestral Medicine), by Wú Qiān *et al.*	• Famous Qīng Dynasty compendium of medicine • Detailed discussion of psoriasis as an independent disease • "Pine skin tinea is named after the resemblance of the red and white dotted skin of pine tree bark. Itching is constant. *Bái bǐ* arises from the dry white skin as itchy macula and scabs. The scaly white skin is due to scratching. This condition is caused by malnourishment of the skin when blood dryness is caused by attack of the skin by pathogenic wind"[7] • Proposed treatment: oral intake of *Fáng Fēng Tōng Shèng Wán* (Ledebouriella Powder That Sagely Unblocks),[8] *Sōu Fēng Shùn Qì Wán* (Track Down Wind and Smooth the Flow of Qi Pill), and external application of swine fat and apricot kernel powder
Qīng Dynasty 1742	*Wài Kē Xīn Fǎ* (Essential Teachings on External Medicine), written by Xuē Jǐ	• "The skin lesion of psoriasis looks like measles and scabies. The lesions are white and itching"[9] • Main pathogenesis: invasion of wind in external skin • Exterior skin lacks nourishment due to blood deficiency (*xuè xū* 血虚)
Late Qīng Dynasty 1831	*Wài Kē Zhèng Zhì Quán Shū* (Complete Book of Patterns and Treatments in External Medicine), by Xǔ Kèchāng	• *Bái bǐ*, also known as *bǐ fēng* 疕风 (wind *bǐ*), various manifestations • Starts with dry and itchy skin, whitish measles- and scabies-like lesions with silver scales • Then generally develops dry and cracking skin all over the extremities and trunk due to lack of nourishment • Bleeding, thickened, and itching skin between fingers, and patient feels constant need to scratch • Often seen in the blood deficiency type

All in all, ancient concepts in TCM already understood the pathogenesis and manifestation of psoriasis to be the combination of internal and external pathogenic factors. External pathogenic factors are mainly summarized as "wind," "dryness," "heat," and "toxin." Modern TCM mainly refers to the pathogenesis of psoriasis as blood heat, subsequently developing into blood dryness and blood stasis, heat, or fire toxin. The major issue in conventional medicine is that all stages, appearances, and types of the disease are treated with the same medication, whereas TCM offers multiple options. One big advantage of TCM is that it allows for an individual treatment, fully adapted to each individual patient's needs. It can treat different stages and different sub-types according to their appearance, caused by different pathogenic factors according to TCM. This enables us to work more precisely with the patient, responding to the most minor influences and changes. TCM offers us great flexibility in its application and multiple options that can be employed to treat each type, subtype, and form, while considering various contexts and living situations.

Etiology and Pathogenesis of Psoriasis According to Traditional Chinese Medicine

As a TCM doctor, one has to look at several external factors in the process of diagnosing skin diseases: the location, the clinical presentation, the duration, and the clinical stage, as well as the accompanying symptoms such as itching, burning, scaling, bleeding, and discharge. It is essential to emphasize that psoriasis does not present with one single appearance. Precise differentiation is very important to develop a treatment concept exactly fitting each individual patient. Without this, the treatment will not be effective, as the same therapeutic principle is not suitable for each patient. This is why, before looking at different treatment options, we need to review the differentiation of location and clinical presentation of psoriasis.

Differentiation of Psoriasis According to the Location of the Lesions

The appearance of psoriasis is different in each case. Psoriasis can occur on any part of the body, either restricted to one location or appearing in multiple locations at the same time. Plaque psoriasis, which is the most common type, typically affects the outside of the elbows, knees, or scalp. But it can also be generalized, which means that the erythema develops into a general redness of the skin, and then becomes erythroderma such as in the erythrodermic type of psoriasis.

However, in general the lesions of psoriasis tend to develop on the lateral parts of the limbs, and especially on the lateral side of the elbows and knees, which mainly comprise the "yáng area." As psoriasis often results from heat evil, the yáng side or the external skin parts are commonly affected. The skin lesions may also concentrate on the torso and scalp. As for the "inverse type," the lesions mostly occur in the intertriginous regions of the skin folds, which is called the "yīn area."

Pictures for each individual location as described below are added for illustration. However, it must be said that some localizations, such as the eyelids, are very rarely seen in clinic, so there are few pictures.

Face (Facial Psoriasis)

Facial psoriasis means one or more persistent, thickened, red, and dry patches on the face. Facial involvement occurs in about half of all patients suffering from psoriasis. Facial psoriasis is usually mild, but it is occasionally very extensive, affecting the hairline, forehead, neck, ears, and, of course, the facial skin itself.

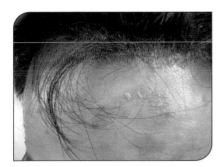
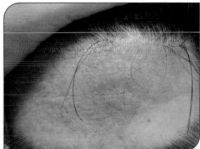

Eyelids

This type of psoriasis is extremely rare. If psoriasis affects the eyelids, scales may cover the lashes. The edges of the eyelids usually become red, dry, and crusty. If the inflammation lasts for a long time, the rims of the lids may turn up or down. If the rim turns down, the lashes can rub against the eyeball and this can then cause irritation and discomfort. It may also impair the patient's vision.

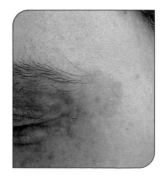

Ears

Psoriasis generally occurs in the external ear canal, not on the inside of the ear or behind the eardrum. Psoriasis in the ears can cause a scale build-up that blocks the external ear canal. This may lead to temporary hearing impairment. Patients often report an accompanying itching sensation in the ears.

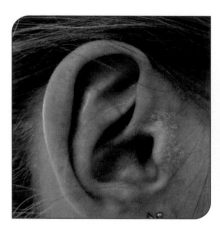 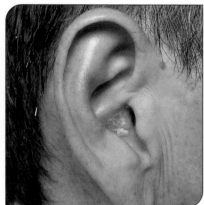

Genital Area

The most common type of psoriasis in the genital region is the "inverse type" (see also above for intertriginous regions of the skin folds, called "yīn area"). Lesions first show up as smooth, dry, red lesions. The following areas can be affected by psoriasis: pubis, upper thighs, creases between the thigh and groin, genitals, anus and surrounding skin, and the crease of the buttocks. In its early stages, this type is often misdiagnosed as syphilis.

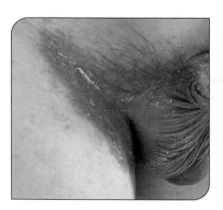 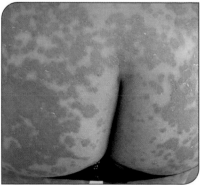

Nails

Nail changes occur in up to 50% of psoriasis patients, and in at least 80% of patients with psoriatic arthritis. The most common nail problems are: pitting, characterized by shallow or deep holes in the nail; deformations, which are alterations in the normal shape of the nail; thickening of the nail; onycholysis (a separation of the nail from the nail bed); and discoloration, creating an unusual nail color such as yellow-brown.

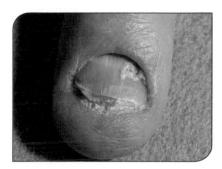 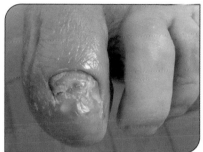

Hands, Feet, Palms, and Soles (Palmoplantar Psoriasis)

Palmoplantar psoriasis tends to be a chronic recurrent skin condition. It involves cracking, blisters, and swelling accompanying flare-ups of acute psoriasis on the hands and feet. Sometimes there is obvious desquamation and pustules. When the palms and soles are affected by psoriasis, they tend to be partially or completely red, dry, and thickened, often with deep, painful cracks (fissures). This condition can be quite hard to differentiate from hand dermatitis and other forms of keratoderma, which is characterized by generalized thickening and scaling of the palms and soles.

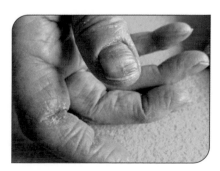 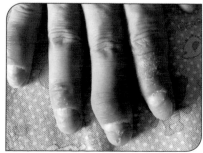

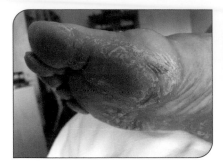 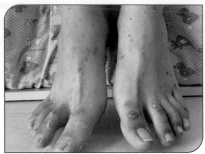

Head (Scalp)

Psoriasis lesions on the scalp can be mild with slight, fine scaling. But they can also be very severe with thick, red, crusted plaques covering the entire scalp. This type can extend beyond the hairline to the forehead, the back of the neck, and often around the ears. Hair loss in patches or tufts is a characteristic feature of scalp psoriasis (*tóu bù yín xiè bìng* 头部银屑病). Because other skin disorders may look similar to psoriasis, it is not unusual for scalp psoriasis to be often misdiagnosed as seborrheic dermatitis or dandruff.

Since hair covers the scalp, patients who suffer from scalp psoriasis at an early stage do not receive sufficient attention in clinics, and medical examination of the lesions is more difficult for doctors. Therefore, these patients are often misdiagnosed. This is unfortunate as psoriasis can persist on the scalp for a long time and only then spread to the entire body. At this point the best moment for treatment has been missed.

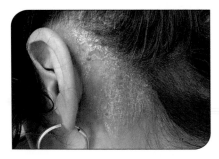 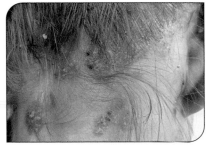

Examples of Other Common Locations of Psoriasis Seen in Clinical Practice

Arms

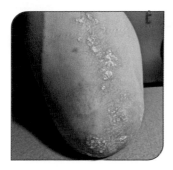
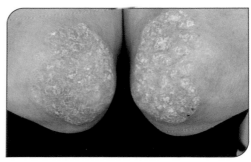

Legs

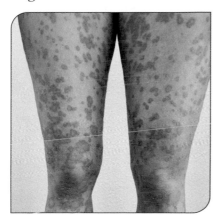
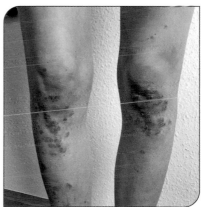

Abdomen

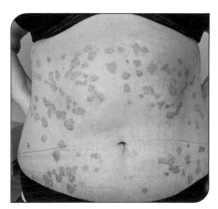
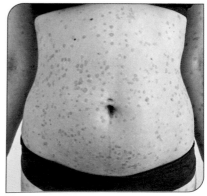

Back

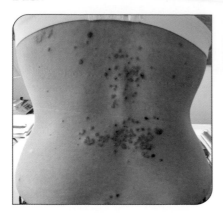 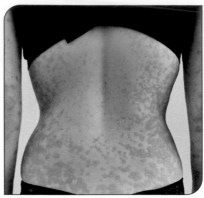

Classification of Psoriasis According to the Clinical Presentation of the Lesions

It has become clear that psoriasis occurs in different locations. What is more, it appears in a variety of forms with distinct characteristics. Typically, an individual suffers from one type of psoriasis at a time. The following provides an overview of the main types of psoriasis, with illustrations of each type to aid in making precise distinctions.

Chronic Plaque Type (Psoriasis Vulgaris)

Plaque psoriasis, also called psoriasis vulgaris (PV), is the most prevalent form of psoriasis.[10]

This type of psoriasis is usually longer lasting than the other types, and is chararcterized by raised, inflamed, red lesions covered by silvery white scales. Lesions are typically found on the elbows, knees, scalp, and lower back. The course of the disease can differ significantly from patient to patient, occurring over many years as a constant infestation or as rapid spreading. Psoriasis vulgaris can be further divided into three different stages: progressive period, stable period, and regressive period.

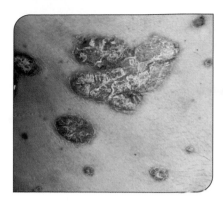
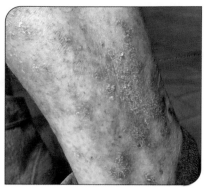

Three Stages of Psoriasis Vulgaris

PROGRESSIVE PERIOD

During the progressive period skin lesions are covered by multilayers of white-silver scaling. Lesions are often irregular; smaller plaques grow into larger ones and merge with one another. At this point one can hardly see any normal skin, as the patient has a so-called skin scale-armor. This is, of course, a very severe form of this type. It is not uncommon for the reddened underlying skin to be completely hidden by the scale-armor when large plaques have merged. The skin is usually very itchy. During this stage, many patients experience the Auspitz phenomenon (xuè lù xiàn xiàng 血露象), blood spots under the scales when their skin membrane is ruptured by scratching something that can happen when patients experience constant itching and cannot help but scratch.

STABLE PERIOD

Stable plaque psoriasis is the most common pattern of psoriasis. It usually begins a few weeks after the progressive stage. During the stable period the persistent plaques tend to appear symmetrically, and any area of the body can be involved. Old lesions are covered with very thick whitish scales, but new lesions do not appear at this stage.

REGRESSIVE PERIOD

During regression the plaques stop growing. They flatten and turn pale, and the scaling decreases. The lesions gradually decrease in size and disappear, leaving a rough surface and discoloration on the skin such as a brownish color of the areas of the skin previously affected.

Guttate Type

Guttate psoriasis is the second most common type of psoriasis, following plaque psoriasis. This type often starts in childhood or early adulthood. This form of psoriasis appears as small, red individual spots on the skin, which look like a "drop." The term "guttate" is derived from the Greek word "gutta," which means "drop." Here, lesions usually appear on the trunk and limbs and they are often not as thick as plaque lesions.

Guttate psoriasis often occurs quite suddenly and is closely connected to typical trigger factors. A variety of conditions can trigger an attack of guttate psoriasis, including upper respiratory infections, streptococcal throat infections, tonsillitis, stress, injury to the skin, and the administration of certain drugs including antimalarials and beta-blockers.[11] In the later course of the disease, guttate psoriasis can turn into a vulgaris type, or can subside if the trigger factors are eliminated.

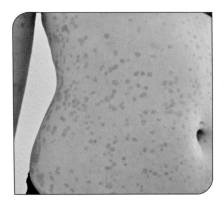 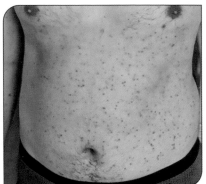

Erythrodermic Type

Erythrodermic psoriasis, also known as psoriatic exfoliative dermatitis, is a particularly inflammatory form of psoriasis that affects most of the body surface. It is a more serious type of psoriasis, which is rarely seen at local TCM practices. Here, the disease often covers more than 95% of the body surface. Known triggers include the abrupt withdrawal of a systemic psoriasis treatment including cortisone, allergic drug reactions, severe sunburn, infection,[12] and medications such as lithium, anti-malarial drugs, and strong coal tar products.

Erythrodermic psoriasis may occur alone or in association with the so-called "von Zumbusch pustular psoriasis." A periodic, widespread, fiery redness of the skin and shedding of scales in sheets instead of smaller scales characterize erythrodermic psoriasis. The patient often suffers from severe itching and pain; the heart rate increases, and a fluctuating body temperature often accompanies the reddening and shedding of the skin. Erythrodermic psoriasis causes protein and fluid loss. The condition may also bring on infections, pneumonia, and congestive heart failure that can lead to severe illness. As this is a severe skin condition, the patient should get medical care immediately. They often require hospitalization, especially in order to prevent the concomitant serious effects mentioned above.

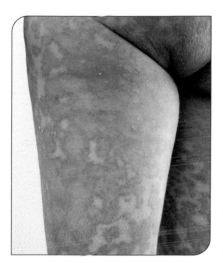 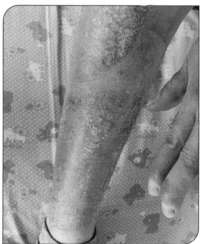

As already mentioned, such patients are usually not seen in a TCM practice. The pictures here provide examples of what the skin can look like; however, the whole body is covered with lesions, with almost the entire skin surface affected.

Pustular Type

Pustular psoriasis is a relatively uncommon type of psoriasis. It is characterized by milky white or canary yellow blisters of non-infectious pus surrounded by red skin, and it is primarily seen in adults. This type of psoriasis may be localized in certain areas of the body, such as on hands and feet, or it can present as a more serious condition, which affects the whole body. It usually begins with the reddening of the skin followed by the formation of pustules and scales.

It may be triggered by internal medication, irritating topical agents, overexposure to UV light, pregnancy, systemic steroids, infections, stress, and sudden withdrawal of systemic medication or potent topical steroids.[13]

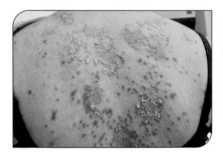 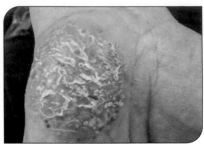

Psoriatic Arthritis

Most patients with psoriatic arthritis (PA) have skin symptoms before they develop joint symptoms. However, sometimes the joint pain and stiffness strikes first. In some rare cases, patients develop psoriatic arthritis without any changes on the skin. It affects both large and small joints. Often the involvement of small finger joints and the knees can be observed.

Psoriatic arthritis usually develops slowly with mild symptoms and it mainly affects young adults. Early recognition, diagnosis, and treatment of PA can help to prevent or limit extensive joint damage that occurs in later stages of this disease. Specific joint damage can be seen on X-ray. Other symptoms of PA include: generalized fatigue; tenderness, pain, and swelling of the tendons or in one or more joints; swollen fingers and toes; and stiffness, pain, and throbbing.

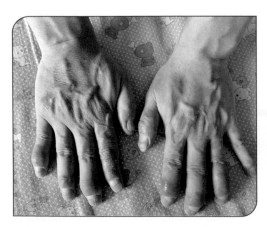 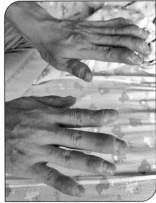

Inverse Type

Inverse psoriasis is usually found in the axillary and inguinal folds, under the breasts and in other skin folds around the genitals and the buttocks. With this type of psoriasis lesions appear bright red. Lesions here lack significant scaling; they are smooth and shiny. Lesions of this type are subject to irritation from rubbing and sweating because of their location in skin folds and tender areas. Inverse psoriasis can be more troublesome in overweight people and/or those with deep skin folds. It is important that the affected areas become less moist. Carefully drying with a hair dryer and weight loss can be helpful.

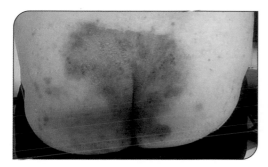 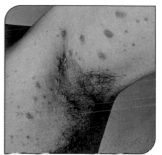

In conclusion, with regard to classification, plaque-type psoriasis is the most common type in our daily practice. Types such as the pustular or inverse type are extremely rare. Even in China, in the big dermatology departments of large hospitals, the plaque type is seen most often. This is also due to the fact that types like the erythrodermic type of psoriasis usually require immediate hospitalization, and so a TCM practice is not the place to find patients suffering from this.

Differentiating Eczema and Psoriasis

Since it is not unusual for psoriasis in its early stage to be confused with eczema or other skin diseases, it is important to know the differences and characteristics of both diseases. If psoriasis is misdiagnosed in its early stages, it becomes more difficult to treat and takes longer to respond. Knowing the differences between psoriasis and other skin diseases such as eczema promotes a correct diagnosis in the early stage.

The following table clearly highlights the differences between eczema and psoriasis.

	Eczema	Psoriasis
Vesicle	Yes	No
Fluid	Yes	No
Crust	Yes	No (only in pustular psoriasis type)
Scaling	+ (normal)	+++ (silvery white)
Itching	+++	+/++
Season	Worse in winter	Worse in winter
Main causes (TCM)	Damp	Heat
Auspitz phenomenon	No	Yes
First onset	Infancy	Later in life
Trigger factors	Seafood, dust mites, stress	Hot food, hot spices, stress, alcohol, tobacco
Stress as trigger	+	+++
Edge of lesions	Unclear	Clear
	Acute, sub-acute, chronic; there are symptom-free intervals	Progressive and latent phases alternating; the patient is rarely without lesions
Location	Mostly in the yīn area according to TCM	Yáng area (excluding inverse psoriasis type) according to TCM

The Relationship Between Psoriasis and the Functional Disorder of Organs and Channels in Traditional Chinese Medicine

We now move on to the complex functions of the organs in TCM, examining which processes can cause imbalances and how the skin changes accordingly.

Zàng fǔ 脏腑 organ theory illustrates the physiologically holistic relationship of the *zàng* organs with the *fǔ* organs. Moreover, it integrates their configuration, constitution, emotions, and the principle of the *zàng* organs in relation to the five seasons. Inner processes of *zàng fǔ* organs manifest externally and, vice versa, external factors can affect the internal organs. It is essential to study their anatomy, physiology, and pathology as well to be aware of the interrelationships between the organs themselves. The following presents an overview of the physiological functions of the five *zàng* organs, as well as of the processes that can cause imbalances and how the skin changes in response. As *fǔ* organs play a subordinate role here, they are not described in detail.

Liver (*Gān* 肝)

According to the five elements, the Liver is associated with the phase wood and its season is spring. The Liver organ stores blood; it is in charge of the tendons, planning, and strategy, while the Gallbladder is in charge of decision making. It manifests in the nails, opens in the eyes, and is the home of the *hún* 魂[14] spirit. The *Huáng Dì Nèi Jīng* (The Inner Canon of the Yellow Emperor) says: "*Hún* is what follows *shén* 神[15] going in and out." Expansion and an innate desire to be straight is the nature of wood.

Considering the expanding nature of wood, the Liver likes a smooth flow of qì within the body. As long as the flow of Liver qì is not impeded, all blood vessels will remain open and unobstructed. Liver qì stagnation can easily arise from a number of causes. One of the main causes is emotional problems or excessive emotions. This means that a person is either experiencing his or her emotions too intensely or, to the contrary, repressing them. Emotional disturbances and disorders such as depression or violent anger or rage can impede the function of the Liver in regulating the flow of qì. The Liver qì becomes superabundant as it is overstimulated when not flowing properly. As a result, this will cause the Liver qì to ascend or, most likely, to stagnate. Blocked Liver qì that cannot move freely and stagnates for a long time within the body produces heat, and if this continues for too long, it gradually turns to fire. It may even cause blood stagnation. Fire consumes yīn and/or blood and affects the Kidneys, resulting in a hyperactivity of fire due to a deficiency of yīn. This can become a vicious circle. Once the Liver is impeded–no matter what the initial trigger is–the person will be more vulnerable to feel anger. The increased anger or rage will further harm the Liver, which results in more anger or rage, which then further damages the Liver, and this can go on and on.

All this results in changes related to the counter-flow of ascending Liver qì. The key manifestations are almost always symptoms presenting in the upper part of the body. With regard to psoriasis, this means that the head (scalp) will most likely be affected first. Psoriasis often worsens after anger, and anger always causes the qì to ascend. Red psoriasis lesions will be observed on the pathway of the Liver channel in an upward direction–an aspect we will return to later. The key to treating the Liver therefore is to first and foremost protect it from anger.

Heart (Xīn 心)

The Heart is the "emperor" of the human body and the major organ networks. Its nature is fire and its season is summer. The Heart is in charge of blood (transformed from *jīng* 精 essence) and controls the vessels and circulates qi and blood. It contains *shén* 神 (spirit) and it reflects on the face and opens into the tongue.

Emotional imbalances such as chronic anxiety, hot temper, passion, tremendous emotional sorrow, or a sudden emotional shock can lead to Heart fire. Irregular sleep and an improper diet can have the same effect. As the Heart is already associated with the fire element, Heart fire is literally fire upon fire. Symptoms like restlessness, insomnia, confusion, delirious talk, or loss of consciousness may occur. If exuberant Heart fire is complicated by an invasion of wind-heat, this will lead to a transformation into heat toxins, which will gradually enter the *yíng* 营 (nutritive) and *xuè* 血 (blood) levels to consume yīn (blood) and body fluids (*jīn yè* 津液). Blood becomes deficient, and therefore nourishment of the skin and flesh will be impeded and the *shén* will be disturbed.

With regard to psoriasis, this means that exuberant Heart fire can lead to a worsening of the lesions, which become bright red. This mechanism can be initiated by a lack of sleep–for example, due to night shifts or going to bed very late, which can be seen very frequently in Western countries. Early bedtime seems to be considered more important on the Asian continent, which might be due to a deeper understanding of living with nature and staying mentally stable and healthy. Sufficient sleep, including bedtime, is very important because of regeneration processes and rest. The body simply needs the time spent sleeping in order to recover.

Spleen (Pí 脾)

The Spleen is associated with the element earth and late summer. It is the postnatal base of life-sustaining energy and is in charge of the transformation and distribution of food essence and fluids, as well as the transformation of pathological dampness. It is also in charge of production of qì and blood, the muscles and flesh, and the extremities. Absorbing and moving are its essential actions, which define the Spleen and Stomach network as the main base of the postnatal energy. The Spleen raises the clear and descends the turbid. Moreover, the Spleen opens in the mouth and lips. Pathologies of the Spleen can be seen in changes of appetite, the sense of taste, or in changes to the gum and lips. The Spleen also prefers slight dryness and has a tendency to become damp (yīn earth) in pathological conditions.

The Spleen contains "*yi*" (意)–the ability to think and remember. Thus, thinking and remembering are physiological activities of the Spleen. Mental disturbances and excessive worry or overthinking, overexertion, or irregular, improper, and excessive diet lead to an impairment of the Spleen and Stomach (*wèi* 胃). As soon as the Spleen and Stomach suffer from damage, food and fluids stagnate and will no longer be transformed. Impaired functions of the Spleen and Stomach can generate qì stagnation and result in internal damp-heat.

With regard to psoriasis, this means that qì stagnation and damp-heat become obstructed in the skin, which in turn creates psoriasis. An exacerbation of psoriasis can often be seen after overexertion and exhaustion, overthinking, or after improper and excessive food consumption with too much fish, seafood in particular,[16] and spicy, fried, and oily food.

Lung (*Fèi* 肺)

The Lungs are the master of qì, associated with the element metal and the season of autumn. The Lungs are very sensitive to the influence of evil qì from outside, because this first enters the body through the Lungs when inhaling and exhaling. Each of the six external pathogenic influences can easily cause an imbalance in the Lungs, as the Lungs are always the first point of contact. The Lungs can also be damaged because of internal factors such as harmful emotions, particularly sadness, grief, and melancholy. Furthermore, the Lungs have an innate aversion, first of all, to heat/fire and wind, but also to cold, dryness, and dampness. In case of impairment due to these influences, the Lungs easily lose the clear and crisp balance and functions of descending and commanding, and as a result of this, the free flow of qì will become obstructed and stagnate.

The Lungs are in charge of the protective qì (*wèi qì* 卫气) and fluids; they are closely related to the skin and hair, warm the muscles and the body's surface, and control the opening and closing action of the pores on the surface. If the Lungs are disturbed and the Lung qì is weak, body hair cannot be properly nourished and becomes rough. An insufficiency of Lung yīn and impairment of the transformation of qì also result in body fluids not being disseminated correctly to nourish the skin and flesh. Due to this malnourishment, the Lungs fail to keep the skin and (body) hair shiny. In the case of weak protective qì, the pores cannot close properly and therefore sweat pours out. This results in symptoms such as chills, fever, and spontaneous sweating. On the other hand, if there is an excess of noxious qì in the Lungs, the opening action of the pores is blocked and the ventilating function of the pores on the surface of the skin is disturbed. Then a disharmony between the *yíng* (the body's nutritive qì) and *wèi qì* with symptoms of inhibited sweating can be seen.

With regard to psoriasis, this means that an acute onset or exacerbation of psoriasis often occurs after a common cold or the flu. In this case, psoriasis is always accompanied by a sore throat. Since it is well known that infections can trigger an exacerbation of psoriasis, it is recommended to ask the patient about an earlier instance of flu or common cold, or a persistent sore throat. The syndrome of wind-heat attacking the Lung channel is very common. It mostly manifests as dot-like or drop-like lesions of psoriasis with significant itching, sudden onset, and a large number of eruptions.

Kidney (*Shèn* 肾)

The Kidneys are the prenatal source or root of life. They are associated with the season of winter. Psoriasis patients with a corresponding family history often show a certain predisposition regarding Kidney deficiency. Of all the organ networks, the Kidneys are located in the lowest position of the body. Their corresponding orifices are the ears, anus, and genitals (the two yīn) and are connected with the Bladder. The Kidneys are associated with the element of water. Consequently, Kidneys are in charge of storing the *jīng* essence, grasping the qì, bones and marrow, and water. They also contain the will. Furthermore, the *mìng mén* 命门 fire is stored between the Kidneys.

The Kidney *jīng* comprises both the Kidney yīn and yáng—that is, the body's "original" yīn and yáng. The Kidney qì is produced by the physical interaction between the two (Kidney yīn and yáng).[17] The functional warming Kidney yáng steams the material Kidney yīn. The Kidney yīn is the material source of all body fluids, which nourish and moisten all organs within the human body. The Kidney yáng is the source of all types of yáng qì within the body, the "engine" behind all warming, generation, and transformation processes. Both yīn and yáng aspects of the Kidneys rely on and control each other. Thus, the balance between both sides is important for all processes within the body and to maintain health. A deficiency of Kidney yīn must affect the Kidney yáng and vice versa. If the balance between Kidney yīn and yáng is disturbed, a variety of symptoms may arise, such as dizziness, tinnitus, weak or sore lower back and/or knees, night sweats, spontaneous sweating, and burning sensation in palms or soles.

The following factors drain energy from the Kidneys and should therefore be avoided or minimized: overwork, a hard-driven lifestyle, multiple pregnancies and miscarriages, sexual hyperactivity, irregular or too little sleep, chronic illness, and stress.

With regard to psoriasis, this means that there may be a genetic relationship between Kidney deficiency and psoriasis, because the Kidneys are the prenatal source or root of life. Furthermore, it has been observed that psoriasis worsens around menstruation and after pregnancy. In both situations the balance between Kidney yīn and yáng is disturbed. The duration of this psoriasis type is usually longer than others. This type may also manifest as psoriatic arthritis with involvement of the joints.

The Relationship Between Psoriasis and the Invasion of Exogenous Pathogenic Factors

According to TCM principles, both internal (endogenous) factors and external (exogenous) pathogenic factors can cause disease. Endogenous pathogenic factors are the result of dysfunctions of the *zàng fǔ* organs. It is different with exogenous factors: they affect us from the outside and can make us sick. This is why we must be wary of the exogenous factors we are exposed to.

Exogenous pathogenic factors are the six variations in the climate of the five seasons, also known as the "six exogenous qì."[18] The six climatic factors are pathogenic wind (*fēng* 风), cold (*hán* 寒), summer-heat (*shǔ* 暑), dampness (*shī* 湿), dryness (*zào* 燥), and heat (*rè* 热) (fire, *huǒ* 火). We all live in this world, constantly in contact with these natural climatic factors (theoretically) depending on the seasons. Under normal conditions, the human body has the ability to adapt to climatic changes and alterations. If the harmonic relationship between human beings and nature is broken, however, the body is unable to adapt to the variations of the climate. This can be either when bodily resistance is too weak or if there are abnormal or unseasonal weather patterns, which exceed the body's ability to adapt. Whatever the cause, the consequence is that in such conditions the six natural climatic factors become pathogenic factors and cause an outbreak of disease. Patients often ask how it can be possible that a strong body or strong immune system can become sick. The answer is that sometimes the external factor is simply too strong to be repelled. There are different mechanisms of getting sick. In a situation like this, it can be helpful to explain the Daoist principle, as the basics of TCM come from Daoism: the human being should be in harmony with nature and the self. If we understand nature, it is easier for us to stay healthy.

In skin diseases such as psoriasis the consequences are clear. Rather than being repelled, these external pathogenic factors settle in the skin and flesh, influencing the normal qì dynamic. They disturb not only the flow of qì but also can obstruct channels and network vessels. If they stagnate in the skin, flesh, or the interstices, the skin and flesh are deprived of nourishment. This malnourishment can cause, for instance, dryness and diminished elasticity or discoloration of the skin. The skin is no longer able to fulfill its normal functions and skin alterations (and, finally, diseases) occur.

These are external factors that can cause disease. Prior to a summary of both the most common internal and external causes and their impact on the skin—with appropriate treatment suggestions for patients with psoriasis—I would like first to discuss the impact of emotional factors to provide a larger context. There is a deep connection between emotions such as vexation, anger, or rage triggered by emotional, intellectual, or physical strain, or caused by events or a specific situation in life, and the occurrence of psoriasis.

The Correlation between Psycho-Emotional Factors and Psoriasis

The holistic approach of TCM understands the human being as the unity of body and spirit. According to TCM theory, emotions are external manifestations of functional activities of the organs, and inversely the qì of the organs is the basis for the generation of emotions.

In general, emotions in themselves do not cause a disease. Emotions are a normal and natural part of our human existence. Only if emotional stimulations and/or changes are too strong, too excessive, or prolonged can they turn into pathogenic factors, namely "endogenous pathogenic factors."[19] Only when coping is not possible does disease result.

The seven emotional (endogenous) factors are closely related to the five *zàng* organs as well as to the circulation of qì and blood. The seven emotions are anger (related to the Liver), joy (related to the Heart), worry (related to the Spleen), melancholy and grief (related to the Lung), and fear and fright (related to the Kidney), and they are constitutional physiological reflections of the human mental state. An ancient saying suggests: "Anger makes the qì rush upward, over-joy makes the qì circulate slowly, grief consumes qì, fear causes qì to flow downward, fright makes qì flow disorderly, overthinking leads to qì stagnation."[20] Asking patients about personal circumstances and their emotional state is therefore an essential part of any first consultation. In conventional medicine, the emotional state might also be taken into account, but it does not receive the same priority as it does in TCM. Moreover, Western medication is not suited to adaptation in response to emotional influence.

Emotions affect the flow of qì–this is the basis for our discussion. The central concept of qì, our vital energy or "life force," plays an important role as an active principle in understanding the interrelationship between emotional factors and our well-being. An unrestrained and free flow of qì allows qì and blood to move harmoniously, and the individual has light thoughts and can enjoy happiness and pleasure. If the free flow of qì is impeded, it directly affects the individual's emotions. There are two mechanisms: strong emotional changes can impair the essential qì of the corresponding organ, and, vice versa, prolonged dysfunction of an organ usually leads to excessive emotional changes.

When considering the relationship between emotions and the five *zàng* organs, the Liver and Heart are of primary importance. Let's take a deeper look at the Liver as it plays a major role in changes of emotions and psoriasis. The Liver governs the smooth and free flow of qì and therefore ensures balanced emotions. When the Liver loses the function of ordering and freeing the qì dynamic, the Liver qì stagnates and inappropriate or excessive emotions will occur. Heat unavoidably accrues as a result of prolonged and/or severe qì stagnation, and later transforms into fire. As a result, the harmonious interaction between body and mind is disturbed. Outbursts of anger are likely, and patients are very easily irritated. On the other hand, extreme anger can also cause Liver qì stagnation. As stated above, it becomes a vicious circle of harm to the Liver, an increase in anger or rage, and yet more harm to the Liver, if the mechanism is not interrupted. This is quite common nowadays due to increased stress factors, overwork, and many environmental factors and our living conditions, including often overlooked noise or air pollution. Silence and retreat are often difficult to find, although they are extremely important in order to keep our inner balance!

There is one particularly important aspect. When talking about the Liver, it seems that the negative attributes are often at the forefront. Yet there are also positive psycho-emotional attributes of the Liver, which can be beneficial to an individual's personality. These positive attributes of the Liver are worth mentioning: kindness, compassion, and generosity. When treating a disease, however, we need to focus on the negative attributes of the Liver: anger, irritability, frustration, jealousy, rage, and even depression. The term "anger" (*nù* 怒) is rather open to interpretation and can serve as an umbrella term.

Many similar conditions are related, such as suppressed emotion, frustration, rage, indignation, or bitterness. "Anger" is very powerful in a negative sense. And as it is so powerful, it can severely impact and damage the qì dynamic.

Negative Impacts of Excessive Emotions on the Skin

Skin diseases significantly worsen in connection to negative emotions. And, vice versa, the condition of the skin improves as soon as the patient's emotional state improves.

TCM considers the main cause of psoriasis to be heat. Long-lasting anger usually disrupts the up- and down-bearing qì dynamic; qì becomes constrained and stagnant, and eventually transmutes into heat and fire, as discussed previously. Heat and fire lie along a continuum and differ only in their severity, with heat at the mild end and fire at the more extreme end.[21] Since rapid movements characterize pathogenic heat, symptoms caused by heat are characterized by an acute onset and rapid transmission. This can be frequently observed in patients with psoriasis who have an episode of severe stress or periods of recurring angry outbursts. Skin lesions develop very quickly and are bright red immediately after a severe incident. It is not uncommon that a patient you have seen the day before looking good comes into your practice with a severe worsening of their skin. Therefore, it is essential to explain to these patients how important regular visits and formula modifications are.

TCM channel theory is important in determining a diagnosis in dermatology, because the channels serve physiologically as a pathway for transportation of qì and blood. In pathological conditions, they can also serve as a pathway for pathological factors such as wind and heat (fire). Based on this theory, it makes sense that skin changes such as red skin lesions or skin inflammation can be seen along the pathway of the affected channel. If stress, overwork, or emotions such as anger are involved, the Liver channel is affected quite often. If this is the case, bright red, hot, and thick skin lesions with scales can be found, especially in the upper regions–the head, face, ears, and eyes–because of the up-rising nature of heat. As the head is the point of convergence of all yáng channels in the body, the most intense skin lesions are frequently located on the scalp. Note that if heat is accompanied by dampness, pathogenic skin lesions are mainly found in the lower parts of the body, around the genital region and legs or feet. When caused by heat, the red skin lesions can be accompanied by a localized burning and itching sensation. The red color, the hot temperature, and burning all indicate excessive heat. Itching is due to internal wind, which is caused by dryness and blood deficiency. Excessive heat consumes the yīn fluids (body fluids) and exhausts qì. The blood becomes deficient and the skin is no longer supplied with moisture. Thus, distinct scaling accrues, which often makes it difficult to detect the underlying redness of the skin.

Psoriasis can also affect the trunk and limbs, but the onset of psoriasis usually starts on the scalp (head) before spreading to other locations on the body. This is why it is so important to cure the disease at an early stage before it can spread. Soothing the Liver will help ensure this. Thus, paying attention to balanced emotions can help improve psoriasis—and also many other diseases! Particularly in our fast-paced societies and times of increasing stress factors, it can be a considerable advantage to slow down, reduce stress, and listen to emotional and physical alarm signals.

Impacts of Excessive Emotions on the General Body

Results of long-lasting emotional disturbances do not just result in changes to the skin. Other consequences can occur in the context of skin diseases or independently. As explored above, excess yáng (heat) as a result of prolonged qì stagnation within the body often leads to symptoms found in the upper part of the body, such as a red complexion and red eyes, fever, restlessness, irritability, insomnia, and headaches. The tongue is usually deep red. red lateral borders on the tongue, a red tip of the tongue, or occasionally red spots on the tip of the tongue. The pulse is rapid. Checking the tongue and pulse is not only an essential part of making a TCM diagnosis, but also provides information about possible other signs the patient did not mention during consultation. In daily practice, patients often add essential information only when somehow reminded of it. Thus, checking the tongue and pulse is very important and a simple indicator for further enquiries and accurate syndrome differentiation, and should be of great assistance.

Liver qì stagnation also impacts functioning of the digestive system, the Spleen and the Stomach. Typical signs of Liver qì stagnation affecting the digestive system are belching, regurgitation, vomiting, and loose stools or diarrhea. If the Liver fails to smooth the flow of qì, qì and body fluids stagnate. This can lead to edema or ascites, which can develop into very serious conditions. And most notably, if Liver qì stagnates for a long period of time, the orderly circulation of blood is also impaired. Thus, patients with chronic diseases that involve Liver qì stagnation often have symptoms of both qì and blood stagnation (stasis). Blood stasis goes deeper and presents with stronger signs, such as a stabbing pain in the chest, abdominal masses, including tumors, and irregular or painful menstruation. Note that in case of blood stagnation, the tongue and pulse condition will most likely present in a different way. The tongue in such a case has a livid (purple or dark) discoloration and/or purplish veins underneath the tongue, or stasis spots. The deeper the blood stagnation, the more signs can be observed. The pulse can be wiry or rough.

Abundant heat usually drives yīn fluids out of the body, resulting in sweating. Thus, heat manifestations are often accompanied by thirst with a preference for drinking cold water, a dry throat and tongue, dark and scanty urine, and constipation due to the consumption and impairment of yīn fluids. When extreme heat or fire enters the blood vessels, it quickens the blood flow and sears the blood vessels. This causes an abnormal flow of blood, which manifests as bleeding, such as hemoptysis, epistaxis, hematuria, ecchymosis, excessive menstruation, metrorrhagia, and so forth.

Endnotes

1   Translated from the ancient book *Yī Zōng Jīn Jiàn* (The Golden Mirror of Ancestral Medicine).

2   This medical text was discovered during the excavation of the Mǎ Wángduī tomb in 1973.

3   Suí Dynasty (581–618 AD).

4   Translated from the ancient book *Zhū Bìng Yuán Hóu Lùn* (General Treatise on the Etiology and Symptomology of Diseases).

5   Táng Dynasty (618–907 AD).

6   Translated from the ancient book *Wài Kē Dà Chéng* (Great Compendium of External Medicine).

7   *Yī Zōng Jīn Jiàn* (The Golden Mirror of Ancestral Medicine) in Liang Jian-Hui (1988) *Handbook of Traditional Chinese Dermatology*, translated by Zhang Ting-Liang and Bob Flaws. Boulder, CO: Blue Poppy Press.

8   Also known as "Powder of Ledebouriella for Dispersing the Superficies."

9   Translated from the ancient book *Wài Kē Xīn Fǎ* (Essential Teachings on External Medicine).

10 Palfreeman, A.C., McNamee, K.E., and McCann, F.E. (2013) "New developments in the management of psoriasis and psoriatic arthritis: A focus on apremilast." *Drug Design, Development and Therapy 7*, 201–210.

11 U.S. National Library of Medicine.

12 www.psoriasis.org.

13 www.psoriasis.org.

14 The ethereal soul.

15 Usually translated as spirit or mind.

16 More background on seafood and how TCM considers the coherencies can be found in Chapter 8.

17 www.itmonline.org.

18 In Chinese dermatology, other exogenous factors are also relevant, including insects, parasites, and toxins (e.g. medicines, food, paints, cosmetics, chemicals). It should go without saying that all these factors are considered to be harmful and contact should be avoided.

19 Other internal factors, which in turn induce disharmony between qì and blood and *zàng fǔ* malfunction, are an improper diet, genetic dispositions, too little sleep, and overstrain.

20 Silverberg, N.B., Durán-McKinster, C., and Tay, Y.-K. (2015) *Pediatric Skin of Color*. New York, NY: Springer, p.428.

21 Yán Shí-Lín, *Pathomechanisms of the Liver* (*Gān Bìng Zhī Bìng Jī* 肝病之病机), p.174.

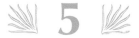

Syndrome Differentiation and Treatment According to Traditional Chinese Medicine

IN TCM, PSORIASIS is caused by an interaction of exterior and interior pathogenic factors (*bing xié* 病邪). Its characteristics can thus be very diverse. Prior to treatment, the exact cause has to be determined according to TCM, by the process of syndrome differentiation (*biàn zhèng* 辨证). TCM syndrome differentiation is the detailed analysis of all clinical information gained by the four main diagnostic TCM methods: inspection (observation), auscultation (listening) and olfaction (smelling), questioning, and palpation. Successful treatment relies on an accurate diagnosis, so the complex process of making a diagnosis according to TCM is essential and cannot be replaced. Although there are root causes and trigger factors for psoriasis, each individual psoriasis patient has a distinctive cluster of root cause and trigger factors. Therefore, every patient presents with a different origin of the disease and suffers from different accompanying symptoms. Each patient is unique, and without precise syndrome differentiation it is not possible to give the patient the proper treatment he or she requires.

The treatment of psoriasis employs various therapeutic methods and combines both internal and external treatments corresponding with the individual clinical manifestation on the skin. In general, psoriasis has to be treated in correspondence with the different stages, first by expelling the pathogenic factors during the active and progressive phase, and then by supporting and supplementing during the regressive (stable) phase. The main patterns are explained in detail below. They are listed according to their frequency of occurrence in my practice and during my clinical studies in mainland China. It should be emphasized, however, that the frequency of occurrence can vary.

The ingredients, functions, and effects of the different formulas used in each individual TCM syndrome as well as their source are listed, elaborated, and explained in great detail. While this primarily serves to increase the understanding for students and beginners, it can also serve as a useful refresher for advanced clinicians.

Heat Stagnation in the Liver Meridian
(*Gān Jīng Yù Rè* 肝经郁热)

It seems to me that the most common pattern nowadays is Liver (*gān* 肝) qì stagnation syndrome with excess heat.

An important role here is played by individual living habits and personal environment. It has been suggested that in over 50–60% of patients, stress and emotional factors, such as anger, are responsible for the onset or exacerbation of the disease. As detailed above, anger and functions of the Liver always affect each other. We have observed in the clinic that psoriasis is markedly worsened after an upset, episode of anger/rage, or stressful situation. Often patients do not report this on their own initiative; therefore, as soon you have the feeling that the patient is in emotional distress, you should enquire after their current circumstances and emotional state. Patients then often confirm preceding factors such as stress or negative emotions before the onset or exacerbation of their skin condition. Furthermore, patients often consume alcohol or cigarettes to cope with stressful situations and overwork, especially young men. Alcohol, cigarettes, and spicy food have been found to be negative factors, which can trigger or worsen heat in the Liver and thus exacerbate psoriasis. Patients also report that lesions get redder and itch more after consuming wine. In women, suppressed emotions as a triggering factor are seen more frequently, because, contrary to the general stereotype, women tend to control their emotions more than men and show them less.

Characteristics

This pattern usually occurs in the progressive stage of psoriasis. Excessive heat and especially upward flaring of Liver fire are extremely complex and lead to numerous clinical symptoms. The upward rising of heat, a yáng pathogen, tends first to affect the head. Thus, the lesions of psoriasis will be most severe at the top of the head and/or on the hairline, and the resulting symptoms on the head can certainly become very intense. Red, hot, and thick skin lesions in varying sizes with scales can be observed, often accompanied by a burning sensation and itching. Itching is due to internal wind, which, again, is caused by dryness and blood deficiency. The skin bleeds easily after scratching, demonstrating the Auspitz phenomenon (*xuè lù xiàn xiàng*). As mentioned above, the lesions can also affect the trunk and limbs, but they mainly start on the scalp.

Other typical signs of heat stagnation in the Liver channel can be a bitter taste in the mouth and dry throat, irritability, dry stool, or dark yellow urine. The tongue is red, which indicates internal heat. The tongue coating may be thick and yellow, depending on the degree of damp-heat present.

The pulse is wiry, rapid, and forceful, which indicates heat excess in the Liver channel.

Treatment Principle

Drain excess heat (fire) from the Liver channel (*qīng xiè gān dǎn huǒ rè* 清泻 肝胆火热) in order to relieve the inflammation on the skin.

Representative Formula

The formula suggested most often is *Lóng Dǎn Xiè Gān Tāng* (Gentian Decoction to Drain the Liver).

Ingredients

lóng dǎn cǎo	Gentianiae, Radix	4–6 g
huáng qín	Scutellariae, Radix	9 g
zhī zǐ	Gardeniae, Fructus	9 g
chái hú	Bupleuri, Radix	9 g
mù tōng	Akebiae, Caulis	9 g
chē qián zǐ	Plantaginis, Semen	9 g
zé xiè	Alismatis, Rhizoma	12 g
shēng dì huáng	Rehmanniae Glutinosae, Radix	15–30 g
dāng guī	Angelicae Sinensis, Radix	9 g
gān cǎo	Glycyrrhizae Uralensis, Radix	6 g

First Reference

Lóng Dǎn Xiè Gān Tāng is a relatively recent formula. The first reference to the formula can be found in *Yī Fāng Jí Jiě* (Medical Formulas Collected and Analyzed, 1682, Qīng Dynasty), written by Wāng Áng. More than 700 prescriptions are listed in this book. The author says that *Lóng Dǎn Xiè Gān Tāng* can clear heat from the organs and he lists the following syndromes where it can be used:

- heat excess in the Liver and Gallbladder
- Liver fire rising
- damp-heat in the Liver.

Formula Analysis

"*Lóng Dǎn Xiè Gān Tāng* cools heat without causing stasis, dispels pathogenic qì and causes it to descend without hurting the normal qì. It is an excellent formula for treating the symptoms and underlying mechanisms associated with Liver and Gallbladder heat excess."[1] It relieves damp-heat from the Liver channel by draining dampness and promoting urination to leach out heat via the lower *jiāo*. The clearing and purging method utilizes bitter-cold herbs, accompanied by nourishing, soothing, and dispersing herbs corresponding with the Liver's yīn nature and its yáng function.

The main ingredients of the formula are: *lóng dǎn cǎo, huáng qín*, and *zhī zǐ*. These three herbs are essential in treating psoriasis. *Lóng dǎn cǎo* serves as chief herb because it accomplishes the primary functions of the formula. *Huáng qín, zhī zǐ*, and *chái hú* are the three deputies within the formula. *Mù tōng, chē qián zǐ, zé xiè, shēng dì huáng*, and *dāng guī* serve as assistants. *Gān cǎo* works as an envoy within the formula.

Lóng dǎn cǎo is extremely bitter in flavor and extremely cold in nature. This makes the herb highly effective not only in purging excess fire from the Liver and Gallbladder, but also in draining damp-heat from the Liver channel. *Huáng qín* and *zhī zǐ* assist *lóng dǎn cǎo* in draining fire and expelling dampness. Bitter herbs such as *lóng dǎn cǎo, zhī zǐ*, and *huáng qín* are usually classified as having a heat-purging effect or a heat-clearing effect. To be precise, *lóng dǎn cǎo* and *zhī zǐ* purge heat and *huáng qín* clears heat from the Liver channel. *Zhī zǐ* is an effective herb for draining the Liver. It also resolves constrained heat and directs damp-heat downwards, leading it out through the urine.[2] In general, it is said that if anger sets Liver fire ablaze, the Liver fire needs to be cleared with herbs like *huáng qín*. In more serious situations, however, herbs that strongly purge Liver heat are needed, such as *lóng dǎn cǎo*. Regarding psoriasis, *huáng qín* on its own would certainly not be sufficient. *Lóng dǎn cǎo* must be added to maximize the fire-eliminating effect.

The Liver, like its associated element wood, has the innate desire to expand and disperse. *Chái hú* disperses heat due to constrained Liver qì. It soothes Liver qì and leads the other herbs to the Liver channel. Since *chái hú* has a pungent flavor, it can directly disperse stagnation. Thus, it is generally recommended for conditions characterized by a stagnation of qì. When it is combined with *huáng qín*, it can clear Liver fire, which is caused by Liver qì stagnation. *Mù tōng* (see caution below regarding the herb's toxicity), *chē qián zǐ*, and *zé xiè* drain heat from the upper burner and remove damp-heat via the urine. As the Liver fire needs a pathway to leave the body, this combination of urination-promoting herbs paves the way. It is an option to remove draining herbs such as *mù tōng* and *chē qián zǐ* from this formula, and thus make it more suitable for treating fire without damaging the yīn as much. If damp-heat increases, these herbs can be returned to the formula. Blood and yīn are easily consumed when fire-heat is in excess in the Liver. Moreover, the components of the prescription are almost all bitter, cold, and drying, and herbs such as *chái hú* also tend to damage the yīn. Thus, *dāng guī* and *shēng dì huáng* are added to nourish and protect blood and yīn while eliminating fire-heat. *Dāng guī* supplements and quickens the blood without causing stasis, while *shēng dì huáng* cools and nourishes blood and boosts yīn. *Gān cǎo* harmonizes the prescription because it mediates the extreme properties of the other components. It tonifies and harmonizes the Stomach, and is used as an envoy and guiding herb in the prescription as it enters all 12 channels.

Lóng Dǎn Xiè Gān Tāng alleviates and improves skin lesions in psoriasis because it eliminates fire in the Liver channel, especially in the upper part of the body. The redder and more severe the lesions on the skin are, the more emphasis should be put on purging fire with bitter and cold herbs such as *lóng dǎn cǎo*, *huáng qín*, and *zhī zǐ*. By purging excess heat in the Liver meridian, the lesions will disappear.

Cautions

Because of their bitter and cold nature, the three herbs *lóng dǎn cǎo*, *huáng qín*, and *zhī zǐ* can easily harm the Spleen and Stomach and should therefore be used with caution in patients with Spleen deficiency or deficiency-cold syndrome. To minimize the bitter and cold character of *lóng dǎn cǎo*, *huáng qín*, and *zhī zǐ*, they can be dry fried (*chǎo*). This method of preparation reduces their cold properties and makes them more tolerable for the digestive system.

Mù tōng, while previously a common ingredient for treating various kinds of skin diseases, has been found to be toxic. The toxicity is due to the herb's aristolochic acid, which is nephrotoxic and carcinogenic. Because of the risk of renal failure and cancer of the urinary tract from prolonged intake and ingestion of large doses, *mù tōng*, as a potential safety hazard, is no longer used and alternative herbs such as *tōng cǎo* are used instead.

Modifications

In psoriasis, heat (fire) in the Liver channel is exuberant and dampness is less prominent. Thus, it is often appropriate to remove *mù tōng* and *chē qián zǐ*. As mentioned above, removing draining herbs from this formula makes it more suitable for clearing heat and fire. One may add *huáng lián* to enhance the clearing action of the formula if it is still not strong enough. Only 3–5 g is required. As soon as the fire is reduced, the dosage of *lóng dǎn cǎo* can be reduced and the herb can be removed later on to protect the digestive system. *Xià kū cǎo* 9 g might be added instead in order to move Liver qì and cool Liver heat. *Xià kū cǎo* travels to the Liver channel and is able to reduce heat in the Liver as well as circulate Liver qì.

For very thick and red lesions, especially on the scalp, add *bái xiān pí* 12 g, *bái huā shé shé cǎo* 10–12 g, or *yě qiáo mài gēn*[3] 12–20 g. These plants are very often used in skin disorders with thick, red lesions. They strongly clear heat and resolve toxicity; they can also reduce abscesses. *Tǔ fú líng* 15–30 g is also frequently used in the treatment of psoriasis because of its cooling and detoxifying effect. For more serious and thicker hypertrophic plaques, add *é zhú* 3–9 g, (*duàn*) *shí jué míng* 30 g, and again *tǔ fú líng* 15–30 g.

For itchy skin lesions, *bái jí lí* 9–12 g can be added. For chronic itching, "wind herbs" often do not work well. "Wind herbs" such as *fáng fēng* and *jīng jiè* are dry and sometimes even worsen the symptoms, because of the dryness and blood deficiency already existing. In this case, herbs that calm the spirit are often more effective, such as *yè jiāo téng* 30 g. Alternatively, *bái xiān pí* 12–15 g can be given to alleviate the itching sensation caused by internal wind. *Bái xiān pí* is very effective in stopping the itching but should be used with caution if given as a single herb or for long periods of time, especially in patients with poor Liver function.[4] It clears heat, expels wind, and dries dampness. This plant is often combined with *quán xiē* 1–3 g to enhance the effect (if available).

The use of *shēng dì huáng* with dosages up to 30 g is very common in psoriasis treatment in combination with *mǔ dān pí* with dosages up to 15 g, especially at the beginning of the therapy. I personally find this combination very effective and use it frequently in clinic. Unprocessed *mǔ dān pí* effectively clears blood heat, but it can easily harm the stomach. Particularly in cases of long-term use of this herb, (*chǎo*) *mǔ dān pí* (dry fried) is advisable, because the cold property has been reduced, but the blood heat-clearing effect is still ensured. Thus, it is more tolerable for the digestive system. In addition, the combination of *mǔ dān pí* and *zhī zǐ* can treat fire due to Liver qì stagnation perfectly. *Mǔ dān pí* is an herb that treats qì at the blood level. Due to its acridity, it disperses and its coolness enables it to drain heat at the blood level. *Zhī zǐ* is a herb that treats blood at the qì level. It clears fire from constraint at the qì level and it also has a blood-cooling effect. Thus, *mǔ dān pí* and *zhī zǐ*, used in combination, can resolve qì-level constraint, leading to heat as well as heat in the blood,[5] as in the formula *Dān Zhī Xiāo Yáo Sǎn* (Moutan and Gardenia Rambling Powder). In addition, if both herbs are used together, they are particularly useful if the patient has psoriasis lesions on the scalp, as a result of ascending heat, which follows the pathway of the Liver channel.

Liver fire often produces headaches and painful red eyes. For these two symptoms, add *jú huā* 9–12 g. Due to its light nature, it can transport the formula to the eyes and head. *Jú huā* and *méi guī huā* are often used in skin conditions affecting the upper part of the body, especially the face or on the hairline. In general, flowers should be considered for the treatment of scalp psoriasis or facial psoriasis. They are light in weight and thus can rise to the head while regulating qì and relaxing emotions. It also helps that patients love flowers and they make the formula look nicer, a useful effect for all patients, not just those "sensitive" to drinking bitter decoctions. All emotional aspects are very important in treating patients with psoriasis. The most suitable flowers to incorporate are *líng xiāo huā*, *lǜ è méi*, *hé huān huā*, or *dài dài huā*.

For constipation, add *huǒ má rén* 9 g. It moistens the Intestine, nourishes yīn, and clears heat. Another alternative for constipation is *huái huā* 9–12 g or (*chǎo*) *dà huáng* 9 g. To protect the digestive system one ought to add (*shēng*) *yì yǐ rén* 9–12 g. (*Shēng*) *yì yǐ rén* protects the Spleen and it can cool heat. An alternative is *bái zhú* 9 g.

For menstrual pain with dark blood and blood clots, add *yì mǔ cǎo* 9 g and *zé lán* 9 g. Both herbs regulate menstruation because they invigorate blood and dispel blood stasis. Moreover, *yì mǔ cǎo* goes to the *chòng* and *rèn mài*[6] as well as the Liver channel, and it is not only cool in temperature but also relieves toxicity. In cases of psoriasis with gynecological aspects, its cooling effects can be employed in addition to its blood-harmonizing effects.

For joint pain, add *rěn dōng téng* 15–30 g plus *jī xuè téng* 15–30 g. This combination is frequently used to stop joint pain and I have had very good experience with this combination in patients with accompanying knee pain. Both herbs soothe the sinews, unlock channels and collaterals, and move blood. *Rěn dōng téng* is able to clear heat and cool blood, which might be required when removing heat in the Liver channel.

A practical hint for taste-sensitive patients with very bitter formulas like this one is to add honey, which makes the decoction a little less bitter and more tolerable. Patient satisfaction is quite important for compliance with Chinese herbal medicine.

Suggestions for External Treatment

1. *Qīng Dài Gāo* (Indigo Cream)[7]

2. *Qīng Dài (Yóu) Gāo* (Indigo Naturalis Ointment)

3. *Pǔ Lián Gāo* (Universally Linked Ointment)[8]

4. *Huáng Lián Gāo* (Coptidis Balm)

5. *Sān Huáng Xǐ Jì* (The Yellow Cleanser Formula)

Examples for individual tailored herbal washes or wet compresses[9] in order to clear heat, relieve itching, moisten the skin, and reduce scaling:

jīn yín huā	Lonicerae Japonicae, Flos	15 g
dì fū zǐ	Kochiae Scopariae, Fructus	15 g
cè bǎi yè	Platycladi Cacumen	15 g

dì fū zǐ	Kochiae Scopariae, Fructus	12–15 g
kǔ shēn	Sophorae Flavescentis, Radix	12–15 g
cè bǎi yè	Platycladi Cacumen	12–15 g
qín pí	Fraxini, Cortex	12–15 g
ài yè	Artemisiae Argyi, Folium	12–15 g

(The second combination can also be used as an external wash for herpes labialis. *Qín pí* may be removed in that case.)

kǔ shēn	Sophorae Flavescentis, Radix	15 g
dì fū zǐ	Kochiae Scopariae, Fructus	15 g
bái xiān pí	Dictamni Radicis, Cortex	15 g
shé chuáng zǐ	Cnidii, Fructus	15 g

Another very simple example of a frequently used and effective combination is this pattern:

huáng bǎi	Phellodendri, Cortex	15 g
huáng qín	Scutellariae, Radix	15 g
huáng lián	Coptidis, Rhizoma	10 g

Please note that other herbs can be added and dosages can be changed as required. For example, *jú huā* or *yě jú huā* can be added if the lesions are in the face. *Jīn yín huā*, *pú gōng yīng*, or *tǔ fú líng* can always be added in this pattern to increase the heat-clearing process and reduce redness and swelling. This combination is often used if the lesions can be found on the upper part of the body, especially in the face. It has been shown to be very effective in practice. More information and standard boiling instructions can be found in Appendix I.

It is also always helpful to inform patients that there are many different possibilities for external applications, and a great variety of combinations. Tell patients that their wash can be adapted very flexibly if needed.[10]

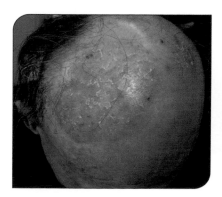
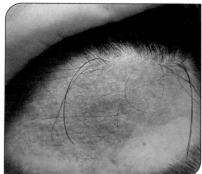

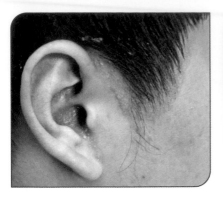 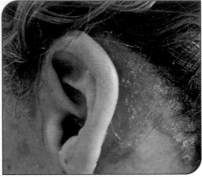

Heat in the *Yíng* Level (*Yíng Fèn Yǒu Rè* 营分有热)

Accumulated heat in the blood is the second most common TCM pattern seen in practice. This is best illustrated by the "four levels" theory developed by Yè Tiān Shì (c. 1667–1746, Qīng Dynasty), which describes the progression of *wēn bìng* (warm and febrile diseases) through the *wèi* (defense), *qì* (qì), *yíng* (nutritive), and *xuè* (blood) levels. However, since psoriasis rarely, if ever, manifests as a *wèi*- or qì-level situation, we will start with *yíng*, the nutritive level, and then move to the blood level to demonstrate the grades of severity and the corresponding changes on the skin. The location of the heat should be determined in order to select the most effective formula for treatment.

Characteristics

When the warm pathogen has passed the qì level, it enters the nutritive level, also called the *yíng* level. At this stage, the disease has nearly reached the blood level, the deepest level. This pattern is very similar to the blood-level stage but is slightly less serious. The nutritive- and blood-level stages are usually associated with the progressive stage of psoriasis. The small skin lesions are bright red. These lesions usually spread on the trunk and extremities, merge, and develop sizable plaques, typically covered with dry, silvery white scales. The skin feels warm and the Auspitz phenomenon can be observed.

When heat has entered the *yíng* level, it scorches and injures the yīn fluids and leads to insufficiency of blood. Accompanying symptoms include slight thirst and high fever that is worse at night. The patient is irritable, restless, and sleepless, because blood belongs to the Heart and consequently the *shén* will be disturbed in this pattern. This disturbance produces mental restlessness and insomnia.

The tongue is scarlet and dry with little coating. The pulse is rapid and/ or thready.

Treatment Principle

Clear heat in the nutritive level in order to eliminate lesions (*qīng yíng tuì bān* 清营褪斑).

Representative Formula

Qīng Yíng Tāng (Clear the Nutritive Level Decoction) is recommended as the representative formula if heat has entered the nutritive, or *yíng*, level.

Ingredients

shuǐ niú jiǎo	Bubali, Cornu	15–30 g
xuán shēn	Scrophulariae Ningpoensis, Radix	9 g
shēng dì huáng	Rehmanniae Glutinosae, Radix	15–30 g
mài mén dōng	Ophiopogonis Japonici, Tuber	9 g
jīn yín hua	Lonicerae Japonicae, Flos	9–15 g
lián qiáo	Forsythiae, Fructus	9 g
huáng lián	Coptidis, Rhizoma	3 g
dàn zhú yè	Lophatheri, Herba	3 g
dān shēn	Salviae Miltiorhizae, Radix	6–9 g

First Reference

This formula originally appeared in *Wēn Bìng Tiáo Biàn* (Systematic Differentiation of Warm Pathogen Diseases, 1798), written by Wú Jū-Tōng (Wú Táng).

Formula Analysis

Qīng Yíng Tāng eliminates heat in the *yíng* level via the qì level by using salty-cold herbs, assisted by nourishing yīn. The original formula contains *xī jiǎo* (Rhinoceri, Cornu). Since *xī jiǎo* is an endangered species, it is no longer in use. *Shuǐ niú jiǎo* is usually used as substitute these days. The situation with *shuǐ niú jiǎo* is similar to that of *zǐ cǎo* in some European countries:[11] while *shuǐ niú jiǎo* is readily available in China, it is not available everywhere.

In this formula, *shuǐ niú jiǎo* serves as the sovereign herb. Since it is bitter and salty in flavor and cold in nature, it can clear heat and relieve toxicity from the *yíng* level. If this herb is not available, alternatives may be required. *Shēng dì huáng* cools blood and nourishes yīn. *Mài mén dōng* has the effects of clearing heat, nourishing yīn, and promoting fluid production. *Xuán shēn* nourishes yīn to descend fire and relieve toxicity. These three herbs used together help *shuǐ niú jiǎo* clear the *yíng* level, cool blood, and relieve toxicity. They protect the body fluids with their sweet and cold nature, and they serve as minister drugs within the formula. *Jīn yín huā, lián qiáo*, and *dàn zhú yè* clear heat and relieve toxicity as well as disperse pathogenic heat. Due to their light-clearing nature, they can eliminate the pathogenic heat in the *yíng* level via the *qì* level. Bitter in flavor and cold in nature, *huáng lián* can clear heart fire and relieve toxicity. *Dān shēn* clears heat, cools and activates blood, and dispels stasis to avoid heat accumulation and blood stasis. The latter five herbs serve as adjuvant herbs. In combination, all the herbs in this formula can clear the *yíng* level, relieve toxicity, eliminate heat, and nourish yīn.

Modifications

In this pattern usually the same modifications are applied as with heat in the blood, as detailed below.

Suggestions for External Treatment

Please see below (accumulated blood heat).

Accumulated Blood Heat (*Xuè Rè* 血热)

As previously mentioned, accumulated heat in the blood is the second most common TCM pattern seen in practice.[12] This pattern is usually associated with the progressive stage of psoriasis.

Characteristics

At this stage, heat has reached the blood level,[13] or *xuè* level, the deepest level. When there is heat in the blood, skin lesions are bright red or dark red and persistent. If the heat is very severe, it can cause stasis and the skin lesions will turn purple. The lesions tend to vary in size and mostly spread on the trunk and extremities, merge, and develop sizable plaques. New lesions continuously appear and, typically, many dry silvery white scales cover the plaques. The skin feels very warm, itchy, and sometimes as if burning. The Auspitz phenomenon can be observed and patients often feel relief if they bleed due to scratching.

Accompanying symptoms can include thirst with a preference for cold drinks and scanty clothing, due to internal heat. The patient has dry stools and dark or reddish urine, and is irritable, restless, and sleepless, as heat is stirring the Heart and the *shén*.

The tongue is deep red with prickles, and the pulse is rapid and wiry or rapid and slippery.

Treatment Principle
Cool and invigorate blood, clear heat, and relieve toxicity in order to eliminate lesions (*liáng xuè huó xuè, qīng rè jiě dú xiāo zhǒng* 凉血活血, 清热解毒消肿).

Representative Formula
If the heat has entered the blood level, the suggested formula is *Xī Jiǎo Dì Huáng Tāng* (Rhinoceros Horn and Rehmannia Decoction).

Ingredients

shuǐ niú jiǎo	Bubali, Cornu	15–30 g
shēng dì huáng	Rehmanniae Glutinosae, Radix	15–30 g
chì sháo	Paeoniae Rubrae, Radix	10 g
mǔ dān pí	Moutan, Cortex	10–12 g

First Reference
Xī Jiǎo Dì Huáng Tāng is originally from the lost text *Xiǎo Pǐn Fāng* (Essay on Formulas, c. 454–473), written by Chén Yánzhī, but the formula is called *Sháo Yào Dì Huáng Tāng* in this book and also appears under this name in the second chapter of the *Wài Tái Mì Yào* (Arcane Essentials from the Imperial Library, 752, Táng Dynasty), written by Wáng Tāo. *Xī Jiǎo Dì Huáng Tāng* as a name for the formula was first used in the 12th chapter of Sūn

Sīmiǎo's *Bèi Jí Qiān Jīn Yào Fāng* (Essential Prescriptions Worth a Thousand in Gold for Every Emergency, 652).

Formula Analysis

The original formula's *xī jiǎo*, or the substitute, *shuǐ niú jiǎo*, and *shēng dì huáng* are the main ingredients in this formula. *Shēng dì huáng*, acting as minister, is also capable of nourishing the yīn and promoting the body fluids due to its sweet, bitter, and cold nature. *Chì sháo* and *mǔ dān pí*, serving as adjuvant herbs, effectively clear heat and dissipate blood stasis if used in combination. All four herbs in one formula have a strong effect in clearing heat, relieving toxicity, cooling blood, and dissipating stasis. If *shuǐ niú jiǎo* is not available, the dosages of the other ingredients should be increased and the formula modified in order to compensate for the effect of *shuǐ niú jiǎo*.

Whereas *Qīng Yíng Tāng* is primarily indicated for heat entering the nutritive level with no blood-level symptoms, *Xī Jiǎo Dì Huáng Tāng* is very powerful for treating heat in the blood level. It addresses symptoms caused by reckless movement of blood and consumed and scorched blood, which can lead to blood stasis. Moreover, it can be seen that the second formula contains no light-clearing herbs, such as *jīn yín huā* and *lián qiáo*, which reduces the "light-lifting" effect of the composition. *Xī Jiǎo Dì Huáng Tāng* works on a deeper level with its blood-cooling and blood-dissipating actions.

Modifications

Chì sháo can be removed if the blood stasis is not severe. If the skin lesions appear purple, indicating that the heat is very severe and has caused stasis, it can be left in. In combination with *mǔ dān pí*, it enhances the blood-moving effect. When the blood has cooled, the bright red color of the lesions disappears quickly. Yet, to reduce the thick plaques, the blood must also be moved. *Mǔ dān pí* is able to perform both actions. To enhance the blood-cooling effect, herbs such as *zǐ cǎo* (if available) 10–20 g or *huái huā* 9–12 g can be added. One should be aware of *huái huā*'s effect of causing diarrhea due to its cold nature and it should therefore be used with caution in patients with Spleen deficiency. If there is heat in the Stomach, the dosage of *huáng lián* is usually 3 g. The dosage may be increased if the heat-clearing effect of the formula has not been sufficient. If the usage of raw *huáng lián* is considered too harsh, the herb can be dry fried (*chǎo*) and thus made more tolerable for the digestive system. If the skin lesions are markedly fresh red, add *bái máo gēn* 15–30 g and *dà qīng yè* 15 g in order to clear heat and cool and regulate blood. *Bái huā shé cǎo* 10–12 g can be added if the lesions are very thick. For joint pain, add *rěn dōng téng* and *jī xuè téng*, 15–30 g of each. The combination of *jī xuè téng* and *dān shēn* is also known to have a very effective blood stasis-transforming action.

Another circumstance that is worth addressing at this point is how to proceed with patients who are vegetarians and/or who do not want to take animal products like *shuǐ niú jiǎo*. If the excess heat is just in the qì level, *shuǐ niú jiǎo* can be replaced by *shí gāo*. *Shí gāo* perfectly clears heat in the qì level, clears Stomach fire, and can be used with dosages up to 30 g. *Shí gāo* is also a viable option in the case of heat in the *yíng* level, but is not suitable as a substitute when the heat has already entered the blood level. In this case, herbs such as *mǔ dān pí*, *dì gǔ pí*, and *shēng dì huáng* should be used at relatively high dosages to tonify yīn and clear heat. Using those herbs in light dosages would quite certainly not suffice. Furthermore, herbs such as *bái máo gēn*, *bàn zhī lián*,[14] and *dù qīng yè* should also be considered to increase the blood-cooling effect. A brief but powerful treatment–that is, using herbs in high dosages especially during the first days of prescription–is advised to relieve the skin. Later on, the dosages can be reduced.

Suggestions for External Treatment

1. *Qīng Dài Gāo* (Indigo Cream)[15]

2. *Qīng Dài (Yóu) Gāo* (Indigo Naturalis Ointment)

3. *Huáng Lián Gāo* (Coptidis Balm)

4. *Qīng Liǎn Gāo* (Clearing and Cooling Ointment)[16]

5. *Rùn Jī Gāo* (Flesh-Moistening Ointment)

6. *Liú Huáng Gāo* (Sulfur Ointment)

7. *Zǐ Cǎo Yóu* (Self-made *Zǐ Cǎo* Ointment)

8. *Yù Huáng Gāo* (Jade Yellow Plaster)

Example for individual tailored herbal washes or wet compresses in order to cool and invigorate blood, clear heat, relieve toxicity, and reduce scaling:

zǐ cǎo[17]	Arnebiae seu Lithospermi, Radix	15 g
shuǐ niú jiǎo	Bubali, Cornu	15 g
shēng dì huáng	Rehmanniae Glutinosae, Radix	15 g

In the blood-heat type, steaming or spraying can also be used, if required. It is a gentler application and not as aggressive on irritated skin. In this case, the herbs are boiled the same way but then sprayed or steamed on the skin.

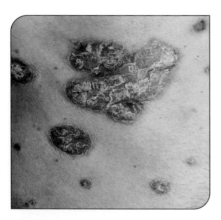
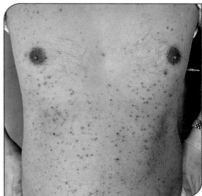
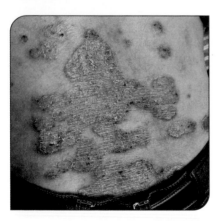
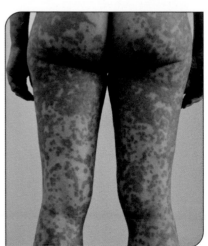

Wind-Heat (*Fēng Rè* 风热) Stagnated in the Skin

Another very common type of psoriasis is wind-heat. This pattern certainly occurs as often as the previous pattern (blood heat). It is not always possible to determine which pattern occurs more often as it varies throughout the year. However, this type usually occurs at an early stage of initial onset or as a subsequent episode after the flu or common cold. This is why it is helpful to ask the patient about a preceding episode of flu or common cold because infections can often trigger an exacerbation.

Characteristics

Skin diseases caused by wind-heat are characterized by a rapid onset, without a fixed location, but with a rapid spreading of many small lesions and itching. External wind-heat (*fēng rè*) stagnates in the skin and in the muscle layer, disturbing the normal flow of qì. It can also obstruct the channels and network vessels, depriving the skin of nourishment, which usually leads to a skin rash with dryness and scaling. The skin is warm, and the lesions are bright red and itchy. This is usually accompanied by an aversion to heat, dark yellow urine, and dry stools.

The tongue has a thin yellow coating and the pulse is floating and rapid, occurring with or without the presence of the Auspitz phenomenon.

Treatment Principle

Dispel wind and release the exterior, and clear heat (*shū fēng jiě biǎo, qīng re* 疏风解表, 清热).

Representative Formula

Yín Qiào Săn (Honeysuckle and Forsythia Powder).

Ingredients

jīn yín huā	Lonicerae Japonicae, Flos	15–30 g
lián qiáo	Forsythiae, Fructus	9–12 g
niú bàng zǐ	Arctii Lappae, Fructus	9 g
dàn dòu chǐ	Sojae Praeparata, Semen	3–6 g
bò hé	Menthae, Herba	3 g
jié gěng	Platycodi, Radix	3–6 g
jīng jiè	Schizonepetae, Herba	6–9 g
dàn zhú yè	Lophatheri, Herba	3–6 g
lú gēn	Phragmitis, Rhizoma	15–30 g
gān cǎo	Glycyrrhizae Uralensis, Radix	6 g

First Reference

This formula originally appeared in *Wēn Bìng Tiáo Biàn* (Systematic Differentiation of Warm Pathogen Diseases, 1798), by Wú Jū-Tōng (Wú Táng).

Formula Analysis

This is a classical formula to release exogenous wind-heat, and it contains many cooling herbs. It clears heat and removes toxins. It is commonly seen in the treatment of the common cold, flu, and upper respiratory infections, but also in various kinds of dermatological diseases such as psoriasis, eczema, and urticaria.

In this formula, *jīn yín huā* and *lián qiáo* serve as sovereigns. Both herbs have the effects of dispelling wind-heat as well as clearing heat in order to remove toxins. *Jīn yín huā* can be used in doses up to 30 g. It is very good in clearing heat from the *wèi* level (defensive level).[18] The first dose of *lián qiáo* should be about 10–12 g to clear heat and resolve toxicity, especially during the first days of prescription. Later on, it should be reduced to 6–9 g. *Lián qiáo* is not suitable for long-term usage because it is very bitter and can harm the digestive system. *Niú bàng zǐ* disperses wind-heat, benefits the throat, and relieves heat and toxins. Together with *jīn yín huā*, *lián qiáo*, *bò hé*, and *jié gěng*, it is used for a sore throat or throat inflammation due to wind-heat. *Dàn dòu chǐ* relieves the exterior. It is good for the early stage of wind-heat with fever and headaches. *Bò hé* clears wind-heat and benefits the throat. The presence of *niú bàng zǐ* in this formula makes it particularly useful for wind-heat that manifests in sore throat, dry throat, and rash. *Jié gěng* and *jīng jiè* dissipate wind-heat and alleviate itching. *Dàn zhú yè*, *lú gēn*, and *gān cǎo* clear heat, alleviate thirst, and generate fluids, and all three herbs are beneficial for the throat.

Modifications

As this pattern is often accompanied by a sore throat, it can be useful to add herbs to treat this. For a sore throat, *dà qīng yè* 9 g and *bǎn lán gēn* 9 g can be prescribed, because in cases of severe heat the formula *Yín Qiào Sǎn* would not be sufficient. Both herbs can reduce inflammatory responses. In the case of a sore throat and diarrhea, it is better to use *mù hú dié* with a dosage of 3–4 g. *Niú bàng zǐ*, which is a component in the original formula

Yín Qiào Sǎn, should not be given when the patient has both a sore throat and diarrhea, because *niú bàng zǐ* is too cold and it moistens the Intestines.

To strengthen the wind-expelling and heat-clearing effects, herbs such as *zǐ cǎo* (if available) 30 g or *huái huā* 9–12 g can be added. Additionally, *bái huā shé shé cǎo* 10–12 g can be added if the lesions are very thick. This herb is very often used in skin disorders with thick, red lesions. It strongly clears heat and resolves toxicity; it can also reduce abscesses. In combination with *jīn yín huā* and *lián qiáo*, it is very often used to treat acute, thick, and fresh red skin lesions. If the lesions are warm and red, *huáng qín* 9–12 g can be added to clear inner heat. The bitter and cold properties of *huáng qín* are relatively moderate compared with herbs such as *huáng lián* or *huáng bǎi*. Thus, especially weakened patients and children tolerate this herb better.

For itchy skin, the combination of *jīng jiè* and *fáng fēng* can also be used, with a dosage of 9 g each. If fever is present, *bò hé* should be decocted within the last 5–10 minutes. If it is used for sore throat, it can be decocted with the other herbs.

Suggestions for External Treatment

1. *Pǔ Lián Gāo* (Universally Linked Ointment)

2. *Qīng Dài Gāo* (Indigo Cream)

3. *Qīng Dài (Yóu) Gāo* (Indigo Naturalis Ointment)

Example for individual tailored herbal washes or wet compresses:

jīn yín huā	Lonicerae Japonicae, Flos	15 g
lián qiáo	Forsythiae, Fructus	12–15 g
pú gōng yīng	Taraxaci, Herba	15 g

Jú huā or *yě jú huā* can be added if the lesions are on the face. *Zǐ cǎo* can be added to maximize the heat-clearing effect. *Bò hé* can also be used as an external application to dispel wind and clear heat. While other herbs are usually given with the same amounts, *bò hé* is usually added only up to 5 g. *Jīng jiè* and *fáng fēng* can also be added to increase the wind-expelling effect and reduce itching. Both herbs applied externally have exactly the same effect as when given internally and can therefore be used analogously.

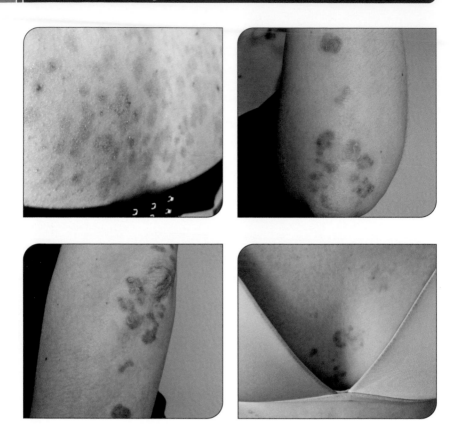

Blood Deficiency and Wind Dryness
(*Xuè Xū Fēng Zào* 血虚风燥)

This is a chronic progression of the disease where the patient has a weak constitution, with deficiency of qì and blood or yīn and blood. Due to blood deficiency, wind is generated, which then transforms into dryness. The skin cannot be properly nourished and becomes dry and rough. An excess of wind results in pruritus (itching) and then in scaling.

Characteristics

The condition is usually stable with no enlargement of the lesions. Lesions are not bright red, but more of a dark red, brownish red, or pale red. They mostly appear as patches or rings. The skin is very dry, cracks easily, and–highly significant for this type–is covered by many dry, silvery white scales. Itching may be slight or severe, and usually worsens at night. If the color of the skin around the lesion is white, it is also an indication of blood deficiency because blood can no longer nourish the skin. This characteristic is often not easy to see, so keep watching for it if you suspect this pattern.

Accompanying symptoms include irregular menstruation with scanty blood, thirst, constipation, dizziness, and a pale and dull complexion.

The tongue is pale with a normal coating and the pulse is thin and deep.

Treatment Principle

Nourish blood and yīn, calm down wind, and moisten the skin (*zī yīn yǎng xuè, qū fēng rùn fū* 滋阴养血, 祛风润肤).

Representative Formula

Sì Wù Tāng (Four Substance Decoction) combined with *Zēng Yè Tāng* (Increase the Fluids Decoction) because yīn and blood have the same source.

Ingredients
Sì Wù Tāng (Four Substance Decoction)

shú dì huáng	Rehmanniae Preparata, Radix	12 g
chì sháo	Paeoniae Rubrae, Radix	9 g
dāng guī	Angelicae Sinensis, Radix	12–15 g
chuān xiōng	Chuanxiong, Rhizoma	6–9 g

First Reference

Xiān Shòu Lǐ Shāng Xù Duàn Mì Fāng (Secret Formulas to Manage Trauma and Reconnect Fractures Received from an Immortal, c. 846), by Daoist priest Lìn Dào Rén.

Formula Analysis

Sì Wù Tāng is a typical simple prescription for treating blood deficiency while regulating blood circulation. *Shú dì huáng*, with its sweet flavor and rich character, is the essential herb in the formula to nourish the yīn and supplement the blood. *Dāng guī* tonifies the blood and helps *shú dì huáng* enrich the blood, but also promotes the circulation of blood. *Bái sháo* and *chuān xiōng* both serve as adjuvant drugs. *Bái sháo* nourishes the blood and astringes the yīn. Combined with *shú dì huáng* and *dāng guī*, the action of nourishing the yīn and blood will be more effective. *Chuān xiōng* promotes blood circulation for removing blood stasis, which encourages the production of fresh blood.

In psoriasis, *bái sháo* is mainly substituted with *chì sháo* because of its blood-cooling effect. Depending on the lesions, the condition of the tongue, and the desired effect, *shēng dì huáng* or *shú dì huáng* should be used. If the lesions are more of a red hue and the blood-cooling aspect has priority, *shēng dì huáng* is more suitable. If the lesions are pale and the patient needs more tonification, *shú dì huáng* may be used. *Shēng dì huáng* and *shú dì huáng* can also be used in combination, but the dampness-generating effect of *shú dì huáng* has to be considered. Adding a small dose of *shā rén* 3–5 g can counteract this effect.

Zēng Yè Tāng (Increase the Fluids Decoction)

xuán shēn	Scrophulariae Ningpoensis, Radix	9 g
mài mén dōng	Ophiopogonis Japonici, Tuber	9 g
shēng dì huáng	Rehmanniae Glutinosae, Radix	12 g

First Reference
Wēn Bìng Tiáo Biàn (Systematic Differentiation of Warm Pathogen Diseases, 1798), by Wú Jū-Tōng (Wú Táng).

Formula Analysis
Zēng Yè Tāng is a typical formula for increasing the fluids to moisten dryness. *Xuán shēn*, *mài mén dōng*, and *shēng dì huáng* all benefit the yīn and moisten dryness. *Xuán shēn*, with its bitter-salty flavor and cold nature, serves as sovereign drug and enriches the yīn, clears heat, increases fluids, and moistens dryness. *Mài mén dōng* and *shēng dì huáng* act as minister drugs in the formula. While *mài mén dōng* enriches the yīn and moistens dryness, *shēng dì huáng* nourishes the yīn and clears heat. Both herbs help *xuán shēn* to nourish yīn, clear heat, increase body fluids, and moisten dryness.

This formula (with or without modifications) is quite often used for treating skin disorders with pronounced dryness as well as other signs of dryness, such as dry oral mucosa or dry eyes.

Modifications

If required, *shēng dì huáng* can be used up to 30 g. It is recommended to add *bàn zhī lián* 9 g to inhibit the keratinocyte cells, and *hé shǒu wū* 12–15 g to further nourish the blood if *Sì Wù Tāng* is not enough. For itching, which in this case is due to internal wind, add *bái jí lí* 9 g. *Jīng jiè* and *fáng fēng* would not be useful here, as they are normally used in cases of an invasion of external wind, rather than chronic itching due to internal wind. They are drying and may sometimes even worsen symptoms, because of the pre-existing dryness and blood deficiency. For severe itching due to internal wind, replace *bái jí lí* with *bái xiān pí* 9–12 g and *quán xiē* 1–3 g; or change to these herbs after one or two weeks of using *bái jí lí* without a significant result. If accompanied by Liver and Kidney (yīn) deficiency, add *hàn lián cǎo* 9–12 g to tonify both Liver and Kidney while clearing heat.

Suggestions for External Treatment

1. *Qīng Liǎn Gāo* (Clearing and Cooling Ointment)

2. *Rùn Jī Gāo* (Flesh-Moistening Ointment)

Examples for individual tailored herbal washes or wet compresses:

dāng guī	Angelicae Sinensis, Radix	15 g
gǒu qǐ zǐ	Lycii, Fructus	15 g
sāng shèn	Mori, Fructus	15 g
dān shēn	Salviae Miltiorhizae, Radix	15 g

This combination is usually given as an ointment or cream. It nourishes the yīn, invigorates the blood, and moistens the skin. To support the enrichment of the yīn and the skin-moistening effect, *bǎi hé* can be added. *Bái jí lí* can be added to reduce itching.

dāng guī	Angelicae Sinensis, Radix	25 g
zhì gān cǎo	Glycyrrhizae Preparata, Radix	25 g

This combination is usually given as an ointment or cream. It may be sufficient for mild cases, but in general it has to be modified.[19]

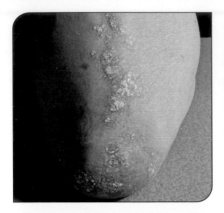
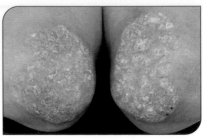
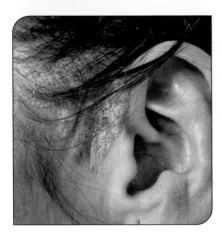
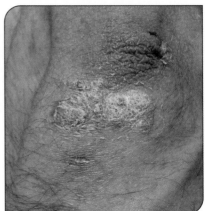

Blood Stagnation (*Xuè Yū* 血瘀)

This is a protracted illness. The flow of qì and blood is impeded and the channels and collaterals (*jīng luò* 经络) are blocked. Due to the stagnation of qì and blood, the skin cannot be nourished, which results in big, thick, hard, dark purplish lesions with chronic plaques.

Characteristics

This is a chronic stage with a long history, and a lot of signs of wear and tear can be seen, such as cataracts and joint pain. Lesions are dark purplish, hard, and thick, and covered by thick, dry, and relatively adherent silvery white scales. The lesions are usually at the front of the leg–that is, the yáng area. New lesions seldom appear. Itching and/or pain may or may not be present.

Accompanying symptoms may include painful menstruation with dark blood and clotting, joint pain, thirst without a desire to drink, and a dry mouth.

The tongue is purple with dark bluish veins underneath the tongue. The pulse is uneven (rough).

One highly relevant observation here is that working night shifts for a long time will always cause blood stasis at some point. It is therefore recommended to check the veins underneath the tongue with patients who work in a profession requiring night shifts. The veins underneath the tongue are usually purplish, which is a clear sign of blood stasis.

Treatment Principle

Promote blood circulation to remove blood stasis, clear toxins, and remove obstruction in the collaterals (*huó xuè huà yū, pái dú tōng luò* 活血化瘀, 排毒通络).

Representative Formula

Táo Hóng Sì Wù Tāng (Four Substance Decoction with Safflower and Peach Kernel).

Ingredients

chuān xiōng	Chuanxiong, Rhizoma	6–9 g
chì sháo	Paeoniae Rubrae, Radix	9 g
dāng guī	Angelicae Sinensis, Radix	12–15 g
shēng dì huáng	Rehmanniae Glutinosae, Radix	12–15 g
táo rén	Persicae, Semen	9 g
hóng huā	Carthami, Flos	6–9 g

First Reference

Yī Lěi Yuán Róng (Supreme Commanders of the Medical Ramparts, 1291), by Wáng Hào Gǔ.

Formula Analysis

Shēng dì huáng, bái sháo, dāng guī, and *chuān xiōng* form *Sì Wù Tāng* (Four Substance Decoction) and together they nourish and regulate the blood and moisten dryness. A detailed explanation of *Sì Wù Tāng* can be found above. As previously mentioned, in psoriasis, *bái sháo* is mostly substituted with *chì sháo* because of its blood-invigorating and blood-cooling effect. *Táo rén* and *hóng huā* both invigorate the blood and transform blood stasis. *Táo rén* is also capable of moistening the Intestines and unblocking the bowels. Therefore, along with its assisting effect in the generation of new blood, it is often used to treat constipation.

Modifications

If the tongue is not pale, the dosage of *hóng huā* should be reduced to 3 g because it is warming. If the tongue is pale/not red, *shēng dì huáng* should be replaced with *shú dì huáng*. For joint pain, add *rěn dōng téng* and *jī xuè téng*, 15–30 g of each herb. To increase the blood-stasis-transforming action, add *é zhú* 3–9 g and *sān léng* 3–6 g. For menstrual pain with dark blood and clots, add *yì mǔ cǎo* 9–12 g and *zé lán* 9–12 g. If cooling action is needed, add *bàn zhī lián* 15 g or *tǔ fú líng* 15 g.

Suggestions for External Treatment

1. *Qīng Liǎn Gāo* (Clearing and Cooling Ointment)

2. *Rùn Jī Gāo* (Flesh-Moistening Ointment)

3. *Yù Huáng Gāo* (Jade Yellow Plaster) (if cooling action is also required)

Example for individual tailored herbal washes or wet compresses:

dāng guī	Angelicae Sinensis, Radix	15 g
sān qī	Notoginseng, Radix	5–10 g
yán hú suǒ	Cordialis, Rhizoma	15 g

These three herbs can be used as the basis for external treatment depending on what else is needed individually. If cooling action is needed, add *bàn zhī lián, tǔ fú líng,* or *pú gōng yīng*. If blood-moving and blood-cooling action is needed, *chì sháo* or *mǔ dān pí* can be used in addition. If there is no pain, herbs such as *sān qī* and *yán hú suǒ* can be removed.

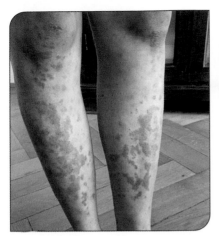

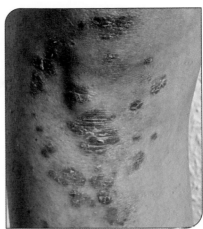

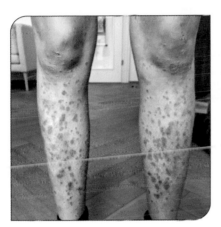

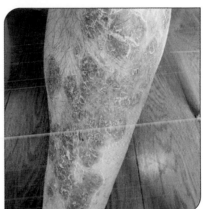

Qì Deficiency (*Qì Xū* 气虚)

This pattern is mostly seen in the stable stage—that is, when the chronic stage and generalized psoriasis has already been treated.

Characteristics

At this stage, the lesions usually fade or turn pale red or reddish brown. Pustules have usually disappeared and there is an obvious reduction in scaling. Accompanying symptoms include lassitude, fatigued limbs, loose stools, and reduced appetite. If the condition worsens after work or doing exercise, this can also hint at qì deficiency. It might be helpful to ask the patient when exactly symptoms or aggravation occurred.

The tongue is pale red, and the pulse is weak or slippery.

A word of advice: in weakened patients with a chronic disease, it is reasonable to ask about night sweats. Do not assume that night sweats only occur in patients with Kidney yīn deficiency. That is a common assumption that does not concur with facts. Night sweats can also happen in patients with blood stasis, or in very weak patients who have been suffering from a chronic disease for a long time. When the disease has prevailed for a long time and the body and the system are too weak to hold the fluids, night sweats can occur. So observe and note all signs and think carefully in order to determine the appropriate treatment concept.

Treatment Principle

Tonify Spleen and remove dampness (*jiàn pí chú shī* 健脾除湿).

Representative Formula

The representative formulas are *Sì Jūn Zǐ Tāng* (Four Gentlemen Decoction) or *Liù Jūn Zǐ Tāng* (Six Gentlemen Decoction), both with modifications.

Ingredients
Sì Jūn Zǐ Tāng (Four Gentlemen Decoction)

dǎng shēn	Codonopsis, Radix	12 g
bái zhú	Atractylodis Macrocephalae, Rhizoma	9 g
fú líng	Poriae Cocos, Sclerotium	9–12 g
zhì gān cǎo	Glycyrrhizae Preparata, Radix	3 g

First Reference

Tài Píng Huì Mín Hé Jì Jú Fāng (Formulary of the Pharmacy Service for Benefiting the People in the Taiping Era, 1107), by the Imperial Medical Bureau.

Formula Analysis

Sì Jūn Zǐ Tāng is a basic formula for treating qì deficiency of the Spleen and Stomach. The original formula contains *rén shēn*. Since *rén shēn* is a slightly warm herb and relatively expensive, when a deficiency pattern is not severe, *dǎng shēn* is usually used as a substitute because of its lower price and neutral character. It goes without saying that in very severe cases and when immediate relief is required, *rén shēn* should be used because it is the most powerful herb to tonify the primal qì of the five organs and it revives from collapse.[20] However, from clinical experience, *dǎng shēn* is quite often sufficient for everyday clinical use, especially in the treatment of skin diseases.

Dǎng shēn replenishes the qì and harmonizes the Spleen. *Bái zhú*, bitter-sweet in flavor and warm in nature, is a key tonic for the Spleen and dries dampness to improve the transportive and transformative function of the Spleen. *Fú líng*, sweet-bland in flavor, removes dampness but it also strengthens the Spleen. This action will be reinforced when used together with *bái zhú*. It also moderates the cloying nature of *zhì gān cǎo*. *Zhì gān cǎo*, sweet in flavor and warm in nature, tonifies Spleen qì and moderates the effects of the other herbs. Combined together, all herbs in this formula tonify the Spleen. When the Spleen qì is strong enough, it is able to perform its transforming and transporting function and eliminate dampness.

Liù Jūn Zǐ Tāng (Six Gentlemen Decoction)

dǎng shēn	Codonopsis, Radix	12 g
bái zhú	Atractylodis Macrocephalae, Rhizoma	9 g
fú líng	Poriae Cocos, Sclerotium	9–12 g
zhì gān cǎo	Glycyrrhizae Preparata, Radix	3 g
bàn xià	Pinelliae, Rhizoma	6–9 g
chén pí	Citri Reticulatae, Pericarpium	9 g

First Reference
Tài Píng Huì Mín Hé Jì Jú Fāng (Formulary of the Pharmacy Service for Benefiting the People in the Taiping Era, 1107), by the Imperial Medical Bureau.

Formula Analysis
This formula is basically *Sì Jūn Zǐ Tāng* (Four Gentlemen Decoction) (explained in detail above) plus *bàn xià* and *chén pí*. It is used when the Spleen and Stomach qì are deficient with accompanying dampness and phlegm. *Bàn xià* dries dampness, transforms phlegm, dissipates nodules, and directs

rebellious qì downwards. *Chén pí* promotes the flow of qì and dries dampness. This formula is usually prepared with the addition of a small amount of fresh ginger (*shēng jiāng*, 3 slices) and dates (*dà zǎo*, 2–3 pieces).

Modifications

In cases of severe Spleen and Stomach qì deficiency, add *huáng qí* 12 g and *shān yào* 12 g. For lack of appetite, add *mài yá* 10 g.

Suggestions for External Treatment

In this pattern, external treatments are usually not required. In order to nourish and moisten the skin, the following combination can be used as an ointment or cream:

dāng guī	Angelicae Sinensis, Radix	25 g
zhì gān cǎo	Glycyrrhizae Preparata, Radix	25 g

Zhì gān cǎo can also be used as a stand-alone herb, then usually given as a cream.

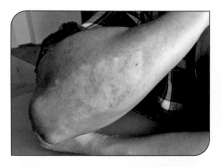
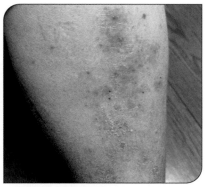
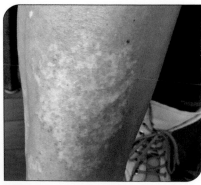
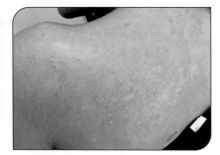

Dampness–Heat (*Shī Rè* 湿热)

While in the excess Liver heat type the heat follows the direction of the Liver channel upwards, it is the opposite case with the damp-heat type. Damp-heat is a pathogenic factor formed by the combination of dampness (*shī*) and heat (*rè*). Dampness is heavy in nature and this will draw the pathogen to follow the Liver channel downwards. The location of the psoriasis lesions and the formation of pustules help distinguish both types.

Damp-heat diseases can be divided into externally induced damp-warmth diseases and internally induced damp-heat diseases. Both categories have different etiologies and signs. Externally induced damp-warmth is caused by an invasion of exogenous dampness together with warmth or a heat pathogen. The body is attacked by exogenous summer-heat and dampness mainly during late summer or early autumn. Moreover, externally induced damp-warmth diseases can also be caused by an improper diet with too much cold, spicy, and oily foods. Internally induced damp-heat is usually caused by a dysfunction of the Spleen and Stomach in their transportation and transformation functions, and an improper diet also contributes to this pattern. As a result, foods and fluids will accumulate in the middle *jiāo* (*zhōng jiāo* 中焦). Chronic retention of dampness easily transforms into heat, and it is often combined with toxins. In skin disorders, damp-heat accumulates in the skin and causes redness and pustules.

Characteristics

Damp-heat is usually seen as erosive erythema (very red and damaged skin) with pustular fluid effusion, itching, and pain. It can affect the entire body with tiny pustules, or only the palms and the soles with local yellow pustules and bright red lesions (pustular palmaris et plantaris). The pustules will vary depending on the predominance of heat or dampness. If there is more heat, the pustules are reddish in color; if there is more dampness, the pustules appear yellowish.

Other symptoms may include a heavy sensation in the chest, loss of appetite, fatigue, a heavy feeling in the lower limbs, or vaginal discharge. Rare but sometimes seen is a yellowish facial color. Note that a yellowish facial color does not only occur in patients with Spleen qì deficiency from a TCM point of view.

The tongue is red with a greasy, yellow coating, and the pulse is slippery and/or rapid.

Treatment Principle

Clear heat and promote urination, clear toxins, and remove obstruction in collaterals (*qīng rè lì niào, pái dú tōng luò* 清热利尿, 排毒通络).

Representative Formula

Bì Xiè Shèn Shī Tāng (Dioscorea Decoction to Leach Out Dampness) if damp-heat is located more in the lower part of the body, especially the legs.

Ingredients

yì yǐ rén	Coices, Semen	15–30 g
huá shí	Talcum	9–15 g
bì xiè	Dioscoreae, Rhizoma	9–20 g
fú líng	Poriae Cocos, Sclerotium	12 g
huáng bǎi	Phellodendri, Cortex	6–9 g
mǔ dān pí	Moutan, Cortex	9–12 g
zé xiè	Alismatis, Rhizoma	12–15 g
tōng cǎo	Tetrapanacis, Medulla	6 g

First Reference

Yáng Kē Xīn Dé Jí (Collected Experiences on Treating Sores, 1806), by Gāo Bǐngjūn.

Formula Analysis

If the lower body is more affected than the upper body, damp-heat has sunken downwards due to the heavy character of dampness. In such a case, a formula such as *Lóng Dǎn Xiè Gān Tāng* would not be sufficient because dampness is predominant, not heat. *Bì Xiè Shèn Shī Tāng* is the best choice if lesions of psoriasis are seen on the legs and the patient shows signs of both damp and heat, because it is formulated mainly for damp-heat diffused downward. The main functions of *Bì Xiè Shèn Shī Tāng* are resolving dampness, clearing heat, and promoting urination.

Yì yǐ rén strengthens the Spleen, promotes urination, and leaches out dampness. It clears heat, expels pus, and clears damp-heat. *Huá shí* also clears heat and promotes urination. It can expel damp-heat through the urine. Topically applied, *huá shí* can absorb dampness from skin lesions. *Bì xiè* separates the pure from the turbid, and consequently resolves turbid dampness in the lower *jiāo* and clears damp-heat from the skin. It is frequently used with *huáng bǎi* and *yì yǐ rén* to treat skin lesions on the lower part of the body caused by damp-heat. *Fú líng* strengthens the Spleen, promotes urination, resolves dampness, and transforms phlegm. Combined with *zé xiè*, it facilitates the removal of stagnant water and leaches out dampness that might be causing edema, swelling, and heaviness throughout the body, particularly in the lower limbs. *Huáng bǎi* effectively drains damp-heat, especially from the lower *jiāo*. It drains fire and eliminates toxicity. *Mǔ dān pí* clears heat, cools the blood, drains pus, and reduces swelling. *Zé xiè* promotes urination and leaches out dampness through the Bladder. It clears blazing ministerial fire in the Kidneys by draining damp-heat from the lower *jiāo*. And finally *tōng cǎo* also promotes urination and clears heat. Because of the cold and draining properties of these herbs, this formula should be used with caution in patients with qì and yīn deficiencies.

Modifications
One can add *qín pí* 6–9 g and *kǔ shēn* 6–9 g as these herbs remove dampness and inhibit cell growth.[?] Inhibiting cell growth seems to be key in treating psoriasis. To enhance the heat-clearing action of the formula, add *huáng lián* 3–5 g. For joint pain, add *dú huó* 6–9 g and *qiāng huó* 6–9 g to alleviate the pain. To intensify the heat-clearing and dampness-resolving effect, add *tǔ fú líng* 30 g. For long-term use it is suggested to use herbs such as *mǔ dān pí*, *huáng bǎi*, and *huáng lián* as *chǎo* (dry fried), making them more tolerable for the digestive system.

Alternative Formula
If damp-heat is mainly located in the upper part of the body, especially on the head, use *Lóng Dǎn Xiè Gān Tāng* (Gentian Decoction to Drain the Liver). *Lóng dǎn cǎo* has a stronger action on clearing heat than *bì xiè*, so *Lóng Dǎn Xiè Gān Tāng* should also be used in case of severe heat and toxin.

The ingredients of *Lóng Dǎn Xiè Gān Tāng* can be found under "Heat Stagnation in the Liver Meridian (*Gān Jīng Yù Rè*)" above.

Suggestions for External Treatment

1. *Qīng Dài (Yóu) Gāo* (Indigo Naturalis Ointment)

2. *Pǔ Lián Gāo* (Universally Linked Ointment)

3. *Huáng Lián Gāo* (Coptidis Balm)

4. *Sān Huáng Xǐ Jì* (The Yellow Cleanser Formula)

5. *Jiě Dú Xǐ Yào* (Detoxifying Lotion)

Examples for individual tailored herbal washes or wet compresses:

dì fū zǐ	Kochiae Scopariae, Fructus	12–15 g
kǔ shēn	Sophorae Flavescentis, Radix	12–15 g
cè bǎi yè	Platycladi Cacumen	12–15 g
qín pí	Fraxini, Cortex	12–15 g
ài yè	Artemisiae Argyi, Folium	12–15 g

kǔ shēn	Sophorae Flavescentis, Radix	15 g
dì fū zǐ	Kochiae Scopariae, Fructus	15 g
bái xiān pí	Dictamni Radicis, Cortex	15 g
shé chuáng zǐ	Cnidii, Fructus	15 g

huáng bǎi	Phellodendri, Cortex	15 g
huáng qín	Scutellariae, Radix	15 g
huáng lián	Coptidis, Rhizoma	10 g

Jīn yín huā, *pú gōng yīng*, or *tǔ fú líng* can be added to increase the heat-clearing process and to reduce redness and swelling.

huáng bǎi	Phellodendri, Cortex	15 g
cāng zhú	Atractylodis, Rhizoma	15 g

This combination is called *Èr Miào Sǎn* (Mysterious Wonder Powder). It clears heat and dries dampness. In this case, the combination should be used as a wash to ensure that exudate can be released. There is a saying: "Wet to wet and dry to dry."

chē qián zǐ	Plantaginis, Semen	15 g
dì fū zǐ	Kochiae Scopariae, Fructus	15 g
huáng bǎi	Phellodendri, Cortex	15 g

This combination is suitable if the lesions are mainly at the external genitals and itching and pain is present. It can be used with or without modifications in order to clear heat, stop itching, and relieve pain.

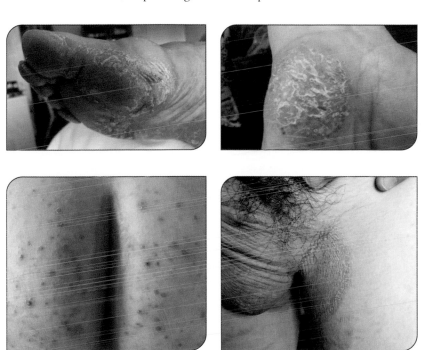

Heat-Toxin (*Rè Dú* 热毒)

In this pattern, severe heat is predominant and it is characterized by an acute onset. Toxic heat accumulates in the body and "simmers" in the skin while redness spreads rapidly throughout the body. Long-term toxic heat harms the yīn and body fluids. The skin feels hot and is covered by scales, which constantly peel off.

This is a severe skin condition. Patients should receive medical treatment immediately and often require hospitalization. I have personally seen a few cases in China, in the in-patient ward. In private practices, this type of psoriasis is very rarely seen.

Characteristics

This is an acute disorder characterized by bright or dark red erythema all over the body, perhaps even a slight swelling, fever, thirst, dry stools, and brownish urine. There is diffuse bright or deep red erythematous skin with, as previously mentioned, characteristic scales that constantly peel off. Almost none of the skin is normal.

The tongue is deep red (crimson) with a thin coating, and the pulse is wiry and rapid.

Treatment Principle

Cool blood, clear heat, and clear fire toxin (*liáng xuè, qīng rè, qīng huǒ dú* 凉血, 清热, 清火毒).

Representative Formula

The representative formula is *Qīng Wēn Bài Dú Yǐn* (Clear Epidemics and Overcome Toxin Decoction).

Ingredients

shí gāo	Gypsum Fibrosum	30 g
zhī mǔ	Anemarrhenae, Rhizoma	6 g
gān cǎo	Glycyrrhizae Uralensis, Radix	6 g
dàn zhú yè	Lophatheri, Herba	3–5 g
shuǐ niú jiǎo	Bubali, Cornu	30 g
shēng dì huáng	Rehmanniae Glutinosae, Radix	10–20 g
mǔ dān pí	Moutan, Cortex	10–12 g
chì sháo	Paeoniae Rubrae, Radix	9 g
xuán shēn	Scrophulariae Ningpoensis, Radix	9 g
huáng lián	Coptidis, Rhizoma	3 g
huáng qín	Scutellariae, Radix	9–12 g
zhī zǐ	Gardeniae, Fructus	9 g
lián qiáo	Forsythiae, Fructus	9 g
jié gěng	Platycodi, Radix	6–9 g

First Reference

Yī Zhěn Yī Dé (Achievements Regarding Epidemic Rashes, 1794), by Yú Lín/ Yú Shī-Yú.

Formula Analysis

This formula is a combination of *Bái Hǔ Tāng* (White Tiger Decoction), *Xī Jiǎo Dì Huáng Tāng*, and *Huáng Lián Jiě Dú Tāng* (Coptis Decoction to Relieve Toxicity). The main functions of this formula are to clear away heat and toxins, remove heat from the blood, purge pathogenic fire, nourish yīn, and stop bleeding. It is very powerful, but sometimes the herbs are still not sufficient. The original formula *Xī Jiǎo Dì Huáng Tāng* contained *xī jiǎo*. Since this is no longer used, *shuǐ niú jiǎo* is used as substitute; however, this herb might not be available everywhere.

Shí gāo and *zhī mǔ* clear heat in the qì level and drain fire, and should be used in large doses. Together they are often used for high fever from wind-heat, heat in the qì level, or excessive heat in the *yáng míng*.[22] *Gān cǎo* clears heat, relieves fire toxicity, and moderates and harmonizes the properties of other herbs, which are extremely cool. *Xī jiǎo, shēng dì huáng, chì sháo, mǔ dān pí*, and *xuán shēn* relieve heat/fire and cool blood. In combination they can remove ecchymosis because of their blood-cooling and heat removing actions. *Huáng lián* and *huáng qín* drain fire and relieve toxicity. *Zhī zǐ* also drains fire and relieves toxicity, and it cools the blood. *Lián qiáo* clears heat, relieves toxicity, clears blood heat, and directs the formula to the upper body. *Jié gěng* benefits the throat and directs the effects of other herbs to the upper body.

If the patient's condition is not severe and he has not been admitted to hospital, it is recommended that the patient stays at home and carefully maintains hydration; however, he still needs to see a doctor.

Caution: The formula is not suitable for long-term use because it can harm the Stomach function.

Modifications

For constipation, add (*chǎo*) *dà huáng* 9 g. For very high fever, *dà qīng yè* 9 g and *bǎn lán gēn* 9 g can be used. If the skin lesions are dark purple, herbs such as *zǐ cǎo* 15 g, *dāng guī* 9 g, or *táo rén* 9 g can be prescribed.

Suggestions for External Treatment

1. *Jiě Dú Xǐ Yào* (Detoxifying Lotion)

2. *Qīng Rè Jiě Dú Xǐ Jì* (Clear Heat and Reduce Toxin Wash)

3. *Qīng Dài (Yóu) Gāo* (Indigo Naturalis Ointment)

4. *Liú Huáng Gāo* (Sulfur Ointment)[23]

5. *Diān Dǎo Sàn Gāo* (Upside Down Powder)

6. *Yù Huáng Gāo* (Jade Yellow Plaster)

These are suggestions for external applications, although, as stated above, these patients are not commonly seen in TCM practices. There are no pictures of the skin or tongue for the heat-toxin pattern.

Summary of Useful Chinese Herbs in Internal Treatment of Psoriasis

Each TCM doctor has their own favorite Chinese herbs. In the beginning, this is because he or she has been taught their usefulness. Later, it will be because he or she has gained positive experience with them. Aside from this, however, various clinical trials have shown the most commonly used and effective Chinese medicinal ingredients in the treatment of psoriasis.

The main herbal substances which have been identified and are frequently mentioned as the ingredients most used in TCM formulas to treat psoriasis are: *shēng dì huáng, dāng guī, dān shēn, bái xiān pí, tǔ fú líng, bái huā shé shé cǎo, zǐ cǎo, chì sháo, bái sháo, hóng huā*, and *gān cǎo*.[24] There are further herbs that should be added to this list. Chinese herbs such as *lóng dǎn cǎo, zhī zǐ*, and *huáng qín* as well as *qīng dài* have not been mentioned in this context in articles and books so far. All of these herbs have been found to have a significant anti-proliferative and anti-inflammatory effect, which seems to be a key function in treating psoriasis, according to modern research. This finding is investigated more deeply in Chapter 6. Also, *mǔ dān pí* is helpful in nearly every patient in the progressive stage of psoriasis. Combined with *shēng dì huáng*, it cools the blood and the lesions fade.

Furthermore, guiding herbs can be added to convey the formula to the affected area of the body. Some examples[25] that have frequently shown good results are found in the following table.

Affected body region	Guiding herb
Face	*jú huā, méi guī huā*
Upper limbs	*sāng zhī*[26]
(Heat affecting the) upper body	*fú píng*
Upper back	*gé gēn*
Lower back	*xù duàn*
Chest	*chén pí, jú yè*
Legs	*niú xī,*[27] *mù guā*

It can be quite useful to add guiding herbs to the formula to send the herbs to body regions that are far from the trunk, such as the extremities and the head.

In this context, we should mention a modern Chinese TCM skin specialist who has done extraordinary work and has created many effective formulas and strategies for the treatment of stubborn conditions such as psoriasis, Prof. Zhào Bǐng Nán.[28] He emphasized for all skin diseases in general: "Although skin disease manifests on the exterior, in reality the core of the problem has its root in the interior. If there is no internal chaos there will be no external manifestation."[29] This statement certainly holds true. Without treating the internal cause, the external manifestation can never be cured. This is also the major difference between conventional medicine and TCM: by treating only the symptoms, no long-term solution can be achieved. This is why patients often report that the skin lesions return after drug discontinuation.

Prof. Zhào worked extensively on creating new treatment options for patients with psoriasis. He advocated the treatment of psoriasis from the "blood aspect." In addressing the blood aspect, Prof. Zhào proposed blood cooling and heat clearing as well as blood moving and transforming stasis with herbs such as (*shēng*) *huái huā, bái máo gēn, shēng dì huáng, chì sháo, dān shēn, zǐ cǎo gēn,* and *jī xuè téng.* Herbs such as *shēng dì huáng, chì sháo, dān shēn,* and *jī xuè téng* are quite often used in practice. According to Prof. Zhào, internal heat and fire are often caused by emotional stress. Emotional stress in turn blocks the free movement of qì. If qì cannot flow freely, qì accumulates and heat (and later on fire) arises.[30] It is well known that when the disease course is long, yīn and blood will be exhausted, which leads to pathogenic wind or blood stasis. At the very end, qì and blood have stagnated, which results in skin malnourishment. Thus, the longer the disease lasts, the more the blood stagnates and wind-dryness symptoms appear.

One famous formula he invented is called Zhào Bǐng Nán's *BAI BI No. 1* (*bái bǐ 1* 白疕1), which consists of *shēng dì huáng* 30 g, *zǐ cǎo* 15 g, *huái huā*

30 g, *bái máo gēn* 30 g, *dān shēn* 15 g, *jī xuè téng* 30 g, and *chì sháo* 15 g. *Rěn dōng téng* 15–30 g can be added if there is additional joint pain (psoriatic arthritis).[31] Zhào Bǐng Nán's *BAI BI No. 1* is a popular formula for psoriasis in its acute, progressive stage. This composition cools the blood, promotes blood circulation, dispels wind, and nourishes the blood.

Another formula, *BAI BI No. 2* (*bái bǐ 2* 白疕2), has the function to cool, move, and nourish blood as well as moisten the skin. It consists of *jī xuè téng* 30 g, *tǔ fú líng* 30 g, *dāng guī* 15 g, *shēng dì huáng* 30 g, *wēi líng xiān* 15 g, *shān yào* 15 g, and *fēng fáng* 15 g.

A personal note: The searchable sources differ partly here with the ingredients of the two formulas. For example, the book *Treatment of Psoriasis with Traditional Chinese Medicine*, by Li Lin,[32] has formulas with the names *Bai Bi 1* and *Bai Bi 2*. However, these formulas are completely different from the formulas found in the book *Zhào Bǐng Nán's Clinical Experience* and mentioned by my professor.[33] With regard to the herbs used, while *tǔ fú líng* and *fēng fáng* can be used in combination to clear toxic heat from the blood, I have personally never seen this combination used to treat psoriasis in China. For this reason, it is advisable not to rely only on the sources you find, which may not be correct in some cases. Draw your own conclusions and learn from your own experiences and apply your results.

Many of the herbs Prof. Zhào frequently used for psoriasis have been common in practice for treating this disease. However, without disregarding the approaches and treatment principles of experts like Prof. Zhào Bǐng Nán, it should be noted that formulas must be modified in our own clinical practice according to each individual's constitution and response, and the stage of psoriasis.

Endnotes

1   Scheid, V., Bensky, D., Ellis, A., and Barolet, R. (2009) *Formulas and Strategies* (2nd edition). Seattle, WA: Eastland Press, p.200.

2   Bensky, D., Clavey, S., and Stöger, E. (2004) *Materia Medica* (3rd edition). Seattle, WA: Eastland Press, p.96.

3   Also called *jīn qiáo mài* (金荞麦).

4   *Bái xiān pí* was involved in a series of cases involving Liver damage in skin disease patients in the UK and New Zealand. An allergic mechanism was suggested. Therefore, this herb should be used with caution in patients with atopic conditions, a history of liver disease and a known poor liver function. Source: Bensky, D., Clavey, S., and Stöger, E. (2004) *Materia Medica* (3rd edition). Seattle, WA: Eastland Press, p.199.

5   Bensky, D., Clavey, S., and Stöger, E. (2004) *Materia Medica* (3rd edition). Seattle, WA: Eastland Press, p.96.

6   Penetrating and Conception Vessel.

7   This is particularly useful for application on exposed skin areas such as the face and hairline as it can be seen in this pattern.

8   Also called *Qín Bǎi Gāo* (*Qín Bǎi* Cream).

9   Boiling instructions and explanations can be found in Appendix I.

10 This applies to all forms and variations of external treatments.

11 Unfortunately, *zǐ cǎo* (Arnebiae seu Lithospermi, Radix) is not available in some European countries. It is a very effective herb and it is used quite frequently in China and worldwide.

12 This pattern often alternates in frequency with the next pattern (wind-heat) according to my practical experience.

13 *Wēn bìng* system: fourth level = blood level.

14 *Bàn zhī lián* is usually used if the lesions are very red. It clears heat, activates blood, moves stasis, and clears inflammation.

15 This is particularly useful for application on exposed skin areas such as the face and hairline as it can be seen in this pattern.

16 Prof. Zhào Bǐng Nán's clinical experience (*Zhào Bǐng Nán Lín Chuáng Jīng Yàn Jí*: Zhào Bǐng Nán's Clinical Experience Set. Beijing: People's Medical Publishing House, 1975).

17 If available.

18 The *wèi* level is typically the initial stage of warm diseases.

19 See the previous combination and its modifications.

20 Bensky, D., Clavey, S., and Stöger, E. (2004) *Materia Medica* (3rd edition). Seattle, WA: Eastland Press; Chen, J.K. (2013) *Chinese Medical Herbology and Pharmacology*. City of Industry, CA: Art of Medicine Press, p.711.

21 This combination can also be applied in *Lóng Dǎn Xiè Gān Tāng*.

22 This pattern is also called yáng brightness disease (*yáng míng bìng* 阳明病).

23 Can also be given as a wash. It clears heat, resolves toxicity, and inhibits inflammation. It is also very useful in the case of bacterial super-infection.

24 Tan, Y.Q., Liu, J.L., Bai, Y.P., and Zhang, L.X. (2011) "Literature research of Chinese medicine recipes for the treatment of psoriasis vulgaris with blood-heat syndrome type." *Chinese Journal of Integrative Medicine 17*, 2, 150–153; Tse, T.W. (2003) "Use of common Chinese herbs in the treatment of psoriasis." *Clinical and Experimental Dermatology 28*, 5, 469–475.

25 Collected information from my clinic hours in China and my Chinese dermatology seminar notes.

26 TCM works in analogies. *Sāng zhī* are the branches of the mulberry tree (*Morus alba*). Arms and legs can also be seen as branches of the body.

27 The name *niú xī* generally refers to *huái niú xī*. Both *chuān niú xī* and *huái niú xī* are capable of guiding the formula to the lower limbs. *Huái niú xī* more strongly tonifies the Liver and Kidneys, while *chuān niú xī* invigorates blood and expels blood more strongly.

28 Professor Zhào Bǐng Nán (赵炳南, 1899–1984).

29 Pearls of Wisdom Seminar in 2012, found at www.pearlschinesemedicine.com.

30 Prof. Zhào Bǐng Nan's clinical experience (*Zhào Bǐng Nán Lín Chuáng Jīng Yàn Jí*: Zhào Bǐng Nán's Clinical Experience Set. Beijing: People's Medical Publishing House, 1975).

31 Taken from my Chinese dermatology seminar notes; Prof. Zhào Bǐng Nán's clinical experience (*Zhào Bǐng Nán Lín Chuáng Jīng Yàn Jí*: Zhào Bǐng Nán's Clinical Experience Set. Beijing: People's Medical Publishing House, 1975).

32 Lin, L. (1990) *Treatment of Psoriasis with Traditional Chinese Medicine* (1st edition). Hong Kong: Hai Feng Publishing (out of print).

33 Prof. Mǎ Lìlì.

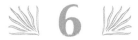

6

Modern Pharmacological Research

THE NEED FOR modern pharmacology and scientific studies as evidence for the efficacy of remedies is a modern phenomenon. But Chinese medicine is evolving and integrates the latest scientific insights to explain the mechanisms and actions of herbs and formulas in a modern way. Chinese herbs and even complete prescriptions with their individual constituents have been examined biochemically. The results are remarkable, though not surprising, and show the complex impact of our Chinese herbs. It could be argued that thousands of years of efficacy does not require further proof, but these modern scientific findings can speak to Western medical experts, scholars, and scientists who have been skeptical about the effectiveness of Chinese medicine. And it may also help expand our own knowledge.

Pharmacological research into Chinese herbs investigates the biochemical or pharmacological properties of medicinal plants and how these properties relate to the chemical, molecular, and physical changes in the body when ingesting medicinal substances. These active biochemical ingredients give the herb or medicinal substance their therapeutic properties. The investigation of the pharmacology of Chinese herbs has been intensive over the past three decades and remains one of the focal points of Chinese medical research in China and worldwide. There has been a tremendous increase in the use and knowledge of Chinese herbal medicine. The major active chemical constituents with a characteristic profile have been identified by analytical methods in lab tests and described in monographs.[1] In addition to this, clinical studies explain the biochemical modes and synergistic effects of components in a clinically proven TCM formula. This research can help to bridge the gap between TCM and conventional medicine, which has become too dependent on the profit-oriented pharmaceutical industry in many instances, demonstrating that TCM offers effective, safe treatment and patient satisfaction.

In psoriasis, these biochemical data not only help explain the mechanisms of action from a scientific perspective to patients, but can also help us, as TCM doctors, in a more targeted application of Chinese herbs–for example, to inhibit increased cell proliferation. Various Chinese herbs are particularly effective for psoriasis considering this modern research and can be used accordingly, provided that these herbs are compatible with the overall pattern of the individual patient according to TCM. The following section lists and explains the most common and most researched herbs in treating psoriasis.

Promising Herbs According to Pharmacological Research

Qīng Dài (Indigo Naturalis)

Qīng dài is effective in inhibiting the growth of cells, so it is often used in psoriasis and in tumor therapy. Qīng dài and dà qīng yè have the same chemical ingredients and are classed as indigoids. Indirubin, an active component of dà qīng yè, inhibits the proliferation of cells by arresting the cells in the G2/M phase of the cell cycle.[2] (The G2/M phase is the pre-mitotic phase where the cell cycle directly precedes mitosis, during which the cell's DNA is replicated.)

Shēng Dì Huáng (Rehmanniae glutinosae, Radix)

The major chemical constituents of shēng dì huáng are iridoid monoterpenes (2.6–4.8%). In addition, immunomodulatory polysaccharides have also been found. Experimental pharmacology has proven anti-bacterial, anti-diarrheal, anti-hepatotoxic, anti-hyperglycemic, anti-inflammatory, anti-tumor, and anti-ulcer activity as well as platelet aggregation inhibition, immunological effects, enzyme-inhibiting effects, central nervous system depressant effects, and hematological effects.[3] Most of the activities are very useful in the modern treatment of psoriasis.

Interestingly, shēng dì huáng seems to possess the same keratinocyte-inhibitory functions as qīng dài. This aspect is also helpful in inhibiting angiogenesis, the growth of new blood vessels from pre-existing blood vessels, which plays a major role in psoriasis. Angiogenesis can be reduced by blood-cooling herbs such as shēng dì huáng and mǔ dān pí. The combination of *shēng dì huáng* and *mǔ dān pí* is extremely effective and therefore very commonly seen in the treatment of psoriasis.

Mǔ Dān Pí (Moutan, Cortex)

Mǔ dān pí has been found to possess anti-inflammatory and anti-microbial (antibiotic) effects.[4] These actions seem to occur because it can inhibit prostaglandin synthesis and decrease the permeability of blood vessels. Paeonol, the major bioactive component of *mǔ dān pí*, possesses anti-bacterial properties. Moreover, the anti-inflammatory action of the herb is related to the inhibitory effects of paeonol on prostanoid synthesis.[5] As psoriasis is an inflammatory skin disease, the anti-inflammatory action is key in the treatment of the disease. The anti-microbial might be quite helpful in preventing secondary infections on affected skin lesions.

Qín Pí (Fraxini, Cortex)

During the progressive phase of psoriasis, an angiogenic tissue reaction occurs, accompanied by an increased local production of growth factors[6] present at elevated levels within psoriatic plaques including insulin-like growth factor-1 (IGF-1). Blood congestion due to increased release of growth factors (e.g. vascular endothelial growth factor) results in thick, erythematous scaly plaques. In this situation, herbs that inhibit IGF-1 can be prescribed. *Qín pí* is one such herb that can inhibit IGF-1. *Qín pí* and *kǔ shēn* are frequently prescribed together to inhibit cell growth. Laboratory tests have confirmed that during the progressive phase of psoriasis the IGF level is always higher. Therefore, it is recommended to add IGF-inhibiting herbs during this phase. Biological studies indicate that the chemical components of Fraxinus species cortex (*qín pí*), leaves, and flowers "possess significant immune-modulatory activities thought to be due to the presence of hydroxycoumarins, secoiridoid glucosides, phenylethanoids, and flavonoids."[7] In general it can be said that from a biochemical point of view *qín pí* seems to be a very helpful plant in treating psoriasis.

Lóng Dǎn Cǎo (Gentianiae, Radix)

The main constituents and essential therapeutically active substances of the genus Gentiana (*lóng dǎn*, an important genus of the Gentianaceae family) are bitter constituents such as iridoids and secoiridoid glucosides (e.g. gentiopicroside, also known as gentiamarine and gentiopicrine, amarogentine, sweroside, and swertiamarin), xanthone, and flavone. In the treatment of psoriasis, one may use the anti-proliferative function of *lóng dǎn cǎo*,[8] along with its pro-apoptotic actions, anti-inflammatory effects, and immunological influence.[9] The main bioactive constituents, particularly useful for psoriasis, are iridoids, flavonoids, and xanthones.

Iridoids are secondary metabolites of terrestrial and marine flora and fauna, and they have traditionally been used to treat inflammation. Studies revealed that iridoids have a wide range of pharmacological activities, including anti-inflammatory, cardiovascular, hepatoprotection, hypoglycemic, anti-mutagenic, anti-spasmodic, anti-tumor, anti-viral, immunomodulation, and purgative effects.[10] Flavonoids are naturally occurring plant-based polyphenolic compounds found in fruits, vegetables, grains, bark, roots, stems, flowers, tea, wine, and so forth. Experiments have shown that flavonoids possess anti-allergic, anti-inflammatory, anti-viral, and antioxidant activities. Through several different mechanisms, particular flavonoids can exert significant anticancer activities including anti-carcinogenic properties and even a pro-differentiative activity, among other modes of action. Certain flavonoids possess potent inhibitory activity against a wide array of enzymes, but of particular note are their inhibitory effects on several enzyme systems intimately connected to cell activation processes.[11] Numerous cell types, including mast cells, basophils, neutrophils, eosinophils, T & B lymphocytes, macrophages, platelets, smooth muscle, hepatocytes, and others, can be influenced by particular flavonoids.[12] Xanthones are phytochemicals such as gentisin, isogentisin, and gentioside that occur naturally in various plants such as exotic fruits from tropical regions, many sac fungi, gentianae roots, and Aphloia species. Xanthones are highly biologically active and they are responsible for the yellow color of the gentianae root. They possess anti-inflammatory properties and beneficial antioxidant properties. The antioxidant functions of the xanthones result in anti-bacterial, antibiotic, anti-hepatotoxic, anti-allergic, and anti-fungal properties of some xanthones. A study showed that the intake of an antioxidant-rich product significantly enhanced immune responses and improved the subject's self-appraisal of his or her overall health status.[13]

Huáng Qín (Scutellariae, Radix)

This plant has also been well researched and many reliable results are available. The major chemical constituents of *huáng qín* are flavonoids, chiefly baicalin (up to 14%), baicalein (up to 5%), wogonin (0.7%), and wogonin-7-O-glucuronide (wogonoside, 4%).[14] *Huáng qín* is very useful in treating psoriasis because of its flavonoids, which enable the plant to have anti proliferative, skin thickness-, and hyperplasia-Inhibiting functions,[15] which is particularly important in treating this disease. Its anti-angiogenic effects are eminently important in treating psoriasis, and anti-bacterial functions may also be crucial in preventing infections on erupted skin lesions.[16] As psoriasis is an inflammatory skin disease, *huáng qín*'s anti-inflammatory effects may also be essential in treating psoriasis.[17]

In sum, *huáng qín* possesses the following pharmacological effects: anti-hepatotoxic activity, anti-inflammatory activity, antioxidant activity, anti-microbial activity, anti-tumor activity, anti-viral activity, central nervous system activity, immunological effects, platelet aggregation inhibition, enzyme inhibition, and smooth muscle effects.[18] The great majority of these effects are essential in the treatment of psoriasis.

Zhī Zǐ (Gardeniae, Fructus)

The Gardenia family contains about 630 genera and 10,200 species. *Zhī zǐ* is the dried ripe fruit of *Gardenia jasminoides* and is the most commonly used species for medicinal purposes. *Zhī zǐ* contains a large amount of iridoid glycosides, which can be linked to the activity of the herbal drug. However, other classes of constituents such as crocins and caffeoyl quinic acids are also present and can further contribute to the activity.[19]

Anti-inflammatory,[20] anti-angiogenic, antioxidant, and anti-tumor (anti-proliferative) properties play a major role in the treatment of psoriasis. The present results demonstrate that *zhī zǐ* appears to be potent in the treatment of psoriasis, as it possesses all these properties.[21]

Jīn Yín Huā (Lonicerae Japonicae, Flos)

The extracts of both the flower and the vine showed an anti-bacterial, anti-fungal, and anti-inflammatory activity, as well as anti-exudative and anti-hyperplastic effects. Intraperitoneal administration in mice increased the phagocytic activity of the inflammatory cells.[22] These actions are known to be essential in the treatment of psoriasis. Anti-bacterial and anti-fungal effects, for instance, are needed in the prevention of secondary infections on the affected skin.

Zǐ Cǎo (Arnebiae seu Lithospermi, Radix)

Zǐ cǎo, mainly derived from Lithospermum species, L. erythrorhizon in particular, contains various chemical constituents such as shikonin derivatives, phenolic and quinonic compounds, alkaloids, phenolic acids, triterpenes, acidic polysaccharides, and flavonoids.[23] Studies of L. erythrorhizon, the active constituents of root extracts, have found anti-proliferative and anti-inflammatory effects in different cell lines and animal models.[24]

Other research showed inhibited proliferation dependent on timing and dosage by promoting apoptosis and blocking cell cycle progression.[25] This is particularly useful as psoriasis is characterized by massive cell proliferation due to an abnormally shortened cell cycle. Another in-vivo study found that shikonin, one of the main chemical constituents, inhibited TNF-α and angiogenesis, and inhibited proliferation, movement, and network formation in endothelial cells.[26] Besides all these beneficial effects, L. erythrorhizon extracts and shikonin have been documented to have skin-protective effects and improve tissue repair,[27] which could be very beneficial to damaged skin in its own right.

Endnotes

1   Official monographs about nearly all Chinese medical plants are available from the European Medicines Agency (EMEA) and the World Health Organization (WHO). These monographs provide a good introduction and a scientific overview on the safety, efficacy, and quality control of widely used medicinal plants.

2   Hoessel, R., Leclerc, S., Endicott, J.A., Nobel, M.E., et al. (1999) "Indirubin, the active constituent of a Chinese antileukaemia medicine, inhibits cyclin-dependent kinases." Nature Cell Biology 1, 1, 60–67.

3   World Health Organization (2007) WHO Monographs on Selected Medicinal Plants Vol. 3. Geneva: WHO, pp.283–295.

4   Huang, K.C. (1998) The Pharmacology of Chinese Herbs (2nd edition). New York, NY: Routledge, p.404.

5   Nadav Shraiborn, Sirbal Ltd., published June 30, 2015, patent citation US9066974 B1.

6   Growth factors are proteins, naturally occurring substances capable of stimulating the growth of specific tissues. Growth factors can also be called cytokines; however, growth factors imply a positive effect on cell division whereas cytokines is a neutral term with respect to whether a molecule affects cell proliferation.

7   Kostova, I. (2001) "Fraxinus ornus L." Fitoterapia 72, 5, 471–480.

8   Matsukawa, K., Ogata, M., Hikage, T., Minami, H., et al. (2006) "Antiproliferative activity of root extract from gentian plant (Gentiana triflora) on cultured and implanted tumor cells." Bioscience, Biotechnology, and Biochemistry 70, 4, 1046–1048; Ogata, M., Matsukawa, K., Kogusuri, K., Yamashita, T., et al. (2011) "Gentian extract induces caspase-independent and mitochondria-modulated cell death." Advances in Biological Chemistry 1, 3, 49–57.

9   Singh, A. (2008) "Phytochemicals of Gentianaceae: A review of pharmacological properties." International Journal of Pharmaceutical Sciences and Nanotechnology 1, 1, 33–36.

10 Viljoen, A., Mncwangi, N., and Vermaak I. (2012) "Anti-inflammatory iridoids of botanical origin." *Current Medicinal Chemistry* 19, 14, 2104–2127.

11 These include protein kinase C, protein tyrosine kinases, phospholipase A2, and others.

12 Middleton, E. Jr (1998) "Effect of plant flavonoids on immune and inflammatory cell function." *Advances in Experimental Medicine and Biology 439*, 175–182.

13 Yu-Ping Tang, Peng-Gao Li, Miwako Kondo, Hong-Ping Ji, Yan Kou, and Boxin Ou (2009) "Effect of a mangosteen dietary supplement on human immune function: A randomized, double-blind, placebo-controlled trial." *Journal of Medicinal Food* 12, 4, 755–763.

14 World Health Organization (2007) *WHO Monographs on Selected Medicinal Plants Vol. 3.* Geneva: WHO, pp.314–327.

15 Kimura, Y. and Sumiyoshi, M. (2011) "Effects of baicalein and wogonin isolated from Scutellaria baicalensis roots on skin damage in acute UVB-irradiated hairless mice." *European Journal of Pharmacology* 661, 1–3, 124–132.

16 Kowalyzyk, E., Krzesinski, P., Kura, M., Niedworok, J., Kowlaski, J., and Blaszczyk, J. (2006) "Pharmacological effects of flavonoids from Scutellaria baicalensis." *Przeglad Lekarski 63*, 2, 95–96.

17 Chi, Y.S., Lim, H., Park, H., and Kim, H.P. (2003) "Effects of wogonin, a plant flavone from Scutellaria radix, on skin inflammation: In vivo regulation of inflammation-associated gene expression." *Biochemical Pharmacology* 66, 7, 1271–1278.

18 World Health Organization (2007) *WHO Monographs on Selected Medicinal Plants Vol. 3.* Geneva: WHO, pp.314–327.

19 Wagner, H., Bauer, R., Peigen, X., Jianming, C., *et al.* (2004) *Chinese Drug Monograph and Analysis. Fructus Gardenia–Zhizi 5 (22).* Germany: Verlagfür Ganzheitliche Medizin.

20 Yunhe Fu, Bo Liu, Jinhua Liu, Zhicheng Liu, *et al.* (2012) "Geniposide, from *Gardenia jasminoides Ellis*, inhibits the inflammatory response in the primary mouse macrophages and mouse models." *International Immunopharmacology 14*, 4, 792–798.

21 Lin, Y.J., Lai, C.C., Lai, C.H., Sue, S.C., *et al.* (2013) "Inhibition of enterovirus 71 infections and viral IRES activity by Fructus gardeniae and geniposide." *European Journal of Medicinal Chemistry* 62, 206–213.

22 Nadav Shraiborn, Sirbal Ltd., published June 30, 2015, patent citation US9066974 B1.

23 Huang, Z.S., Zhang, M., Ma, L., and Gu, L.Q. (2000) "A survey of chemical and pharmacological studies on *zicao*." *Natural Product Research and Development 12*, 1, 73–82.

24 Rajasekar, S., Park, D.J., Park, C., Park, S., *et al.* (2012) "In vitro and in vivo anticancer effects of *Lithospermum erythrorhizon* extract on B16F10 murine melanoma." *Journal of Ethnopharmacology 144*, 2, 335–345.

25 Zhang, Z.Q., Cao, X.C., Zhang, L., and Zhu, W.L. (2005) "Effect of shikonin, a phytocompound from *Lithospermum erythrorhizon*, on rat vascular smooth muscle cells proliferation and apoptosis in vitro." *Zhonghua Yi Xue Za Zhi 85*, 21, 1484–1488.

26 Hisa, T., Kimura, Y., Takada, K., Suzuki, F., and Takigawa, M. (1998) "Shikonin, an ingredient of *Lithospermum erythrorhizon*, inhibits angiogenesis in vivo and in vitro." *Anticancer Research 18*, 2A, 783–790.

27 Ishida, T. and Sakaguchi, I. (2007) "Protection of human keratinocytes from UVB-induced inflammation using root extract of *Lithospermum erythrorhizon*." *Biological and Pharmaceutical Bulletin 30*, 5, 928–934.

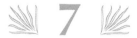

Useful Advice About the Course and Prognosis of Treatment

PSORIASIS PATIENTS in acute stages or with very serious skin conditions must be treated and monitored continuously without breaks. At the beginning, two weeks of taking the herbs daily is recommended. If there is no improvement after two weeks, the prescription needs to be changed, assuming, of course, that the patient has complied with all instructions. If the treatment is followed too nonchalantly, the desired effect will not occur.

Last but not least, it is crucial to inform your patient about the duration of treatment. Again, psoriasis is one of the most difficult-to-treat skin diseases, even in TCM. Be sincere and tell your patient that. Trust is an equally important aspect in the therapy. Chronic and stubborn skin diseases such as psoriasis have evolved over many years and almost all patients have received conventional drugs before, or they are still undergoing treatment when they finally consult a TCM doctor. Thus, instant results cannot be expected, but small changes will occur as treatment progresses. You need to confidently represent your standpoint, because this is the truth. We, as TCM doctors, cannot work miracles in weeks and fulfill expectations that conventional medicine has not fulfilled in 15–20 years, as most adult patients have had psoriasis their whole life. A good and realistic benchmark you can promise to your patients is a minimum of six months of treatment with Chinese herbal medicine. If your patient trusts you, he will be patient in the course of treatment and compliance is ensured as well.

8

Preventive Healthcare:
Dietary and Lifestyle Advice

D IET AND LIFESTYLE habits play an important role in the development of diseases, particularly in the development of skin diseases, as can be observed in clinical practice every day. We know that just as diet and lifestyle habits can worsen a skin disease, they can also improve the skin's appearance. Patients need to understand that they are an essential part of the therapy. They have the ability to speed their skin's healing at home if we create awareness of their own responsibility in their healing process. Or– on the contrary–they may also contribute to the aggravation of their skin disease if they have inappropriate diet and lifestyle habits.

Diet

Chinese food culture, where dining is often a means of promoting communication, is quite different from that in Europe and other Western countries. Eating and hospitability are extremely important in China. One piece of evidence for this is that the greeting formula "Nǐ hǎo!" is often replaced by the question "Nǐ chī guò mā?" which means "Have you eaten yet?" Any host always strives to provide more food than guests can eat, and only the best is on the table.

Apart from the provision and consumption of food, however, Chinese food culture also regards food as medicine. The ancient doctor Sūn Sīmiǎo (581–682) stated: "When treating a disease, nutritional therapy should be used first. Only when no relief can be achieved should medicine (herbs) be used."[1] This statement tells us much about the importance of Chinese dietetics and nutrition, and shows that the combination of nutrition and medicine has a very long tradition.

However, the wisdom of Sūn Sīmiǎo's statement does not seem to be well understood in modern society. This seems paradoxical, as we can observe how popular topics such as healthy eating, yoga, and mindfulness are in the media. It is our duty to educate patients regarding their food consumption and lifestyle habits, and the relationship of these to their individual disease. This is an essential approach because simply prescribing Chinese drugs or giving acupuncture often does not suffice. Without considering and changing these external factors, Chinese medicine treatment is often not enough to treat stubborn and complicated skin diseases. Psoriasis illustrates this very clearly.

Some foods should be avoided and some should be implemented in a patient's daily life if he or she suffers from psoriasis. Some of these recommendations correspond with nutritional advice conventional medicine provides, yet as TCM links foods and effects more clearly, patients will have a greater understanding of how their own actions influence the condition of their skin.

Alcohol, smoking, and oily food have been shown to worsen psoriasis. The effects of alcohol and smoking accumulate over years and decades. They should not be seen in a short-term but in a long-term context. The duration of alcohol consumption, smoking, and bad food habits are proportional to the severity of psoriasis. Alcohol, cigarettes (alcohol more than cigarettes), and oily and spicy food should be avoided in any case. Pepper, chili, curry, onion, garlic, coriander, and other pungent spices or vegetables tend to produce internal heat, so they should be avoided. Excessive consumption of meat and fatty food, which creates dampness and heat, should be avoided. Mild spices, fresh food without additives, fruits, and vegetables should be eaten in their place. Sweet and sugary drinks should also be avoided as they can produce dampness and inner heat. Fresh teas are a highly recommendable alternative for unhealthy sweet drinks.

TCM believes that psoriasis patients should avoid seafood completely. From a modern point of view, seafood such as lobster, shrimp, oysters, crab, or mussels contain high concentrations of purines. Purines are important components of nucleic acids in addition to pyrimidines. Although the mechanism has not yet been fully explained, it is suspected that excessive consumption of seafood can trigger allergic reactions in psoriasis patients. As psoriasis itself is considered an autoimmune disease, it is reasonable to reduce or, better still, avoid the consumption of foreign nucleic acids. In an autoimmune disease, the pathologically activated immune response of the body leads to the loss of tolerance to its own antigens. Too many foreign purines could set off an excessive immunological response, and psoriasis, which was perhaps stable until this point, could be "reactivated." Simply put, there is already an excessive immune system, so do not add fuel to the flames!

From the traditional TCM viewpoint, seafood is classified as *fā wù* 发物. *Fā* means to emit, *wù* means a material or substance. *Fā wù* describes a specific category of foods in Chinese medicine that enhance or worsen disease rather than prevent it, and *fā wù* foods tend to be hot and stimulating. In the case of red-colored skin lesions due to psoriasis, heat is already predominant. When *fā wù* food is consumed, it adds even more heat to the pre-existing heat, and thus makes the skin rash worse. Besides seafood, other *fā wù* foods include chicken and peanuts as well as ginger, lamb, and stir-fried food.[2] They are all warm/hot in nature and have drying properties. These products always tend to generate heat and fire inside the body and injure fluids. This knowledge can be quite helpful in other types of red-rashed skin diseases such as eczema and urticaria.

Patients should have regular bowel movements–at least once a day. Constipation should be avoided as much as possible. If stools are too dry or irregular, the heat within the body cannot escape, which makes the skin worse, as psoriasis is usually a heat-induced skin disease at the progressive stage. It is therefore essential to ask about the patient's bowel movements during each consultation. The patient too should be made aware of how important this is, even if they have come to regard constipation as "normal." If the patient is constipated, it is recommended to deal with this first. Individual tailored formulas will help the patients to regulate their bowel movements. After this is done, one can go ahead with working on the other aspects. Constipation always has to be treated first.

It is unavoidable that different doctors will have different perspectives and dietary recommendations. But no matter which suggestions are given to patients, it is essential for patients to understand the mechanisms behind the food products they are advised to avoid. Knowing why a certain food is not good for them makes it easier for them to follow the doctor's advice. It is also worthwhile noting that we should not be too strict in our recommendations. In my experience, being too strict and dogmatic is counter-productive. Allow the patients to continue to enjoy food, or remind them to enjoy food and not simply consume it, and advise them in more detail along the way. Giving too much detailed information right at the beginning tends to overwhelm, confuse, and stress patients.

Stress and Emotions

Fortunately, the interaction between emotional and mental well-being and physical health are no longer questioned. TCM has always regarded this connection as essential to any healing process. The skin seems to be particularly affected by mental distress and negative emotions. Skin disease in general, and psoriasis in particular, can be seen as a disease of body and mind.

In psoriasis, stress (either occupational or personal) and conflict are often observed as triggering factors. Any full recovery seems to be unlikely without balancing emotions and dealing with triggering stress factors. Patients need to be aware of these mechanisms and pay attention to their emotions and mental health. Patients should be advised to reduce stress and beware of overstretching themselves, both physically and mentally. They need to learn to listen to their emotional and physical alarm signals. A useful guideline for a patient can be the idea that their job should "stretch" them, but not "strain" them. It may be a fine distinction, but patients seem to find it useful in gauging the point at which a useful and healthy level of demand on their abilities becomes too much and begins to create negative effects.

Patients have already been treated with conventional medicine in many cases. As stated above, this most often ends without any permanent success as the disease recurs and may even become aggravated after they cease taking the medication. Patients become frustrated and start looking for alternative treatment options when they begin to realize that the conventional medicine treatment does not treat the root cause. The psychology and mental state of the patient is as important as the treatment itself. As TCM doctors, therefore, we need to explain how our medicine works. We also need to take the time to talk to our patients—and not only at the start of the treatment—because listening is as important as prescribing herbal decoctions.

Lifestyle

The proper handling of cosmetic products and external medicinals is very important. Patients should be advised to handle these products carefully as they can irritate the skin if used excessively or inappropriately. Patients should use "skin-friendly," mild, non-irritating products with little or no perfume. Shower gels should be avoided, as they often contain perfumes and irritating scents, and hot showers are not suitable if the lesions are fresh, red, and hot, especially on the upper part of the body where the hot water comes into direct contact with the body's surface.

Patients should also strengthen their physical constitution, not only for feeling healthy and fit but also to prevent upper respiratory infections. As mentioned previously, it is known that upper respiratory infections, streptococcal throat infections, tonsillitis, and common colds can trigger an attack of psoriasis. Sunlight improves the lesions of most psoriasis patients. Advise your patients to go out in the sun as much as possible as the skin will be very grateful. Wearing shorts or T-shirts can also help to maximize the affected skin's exposure to sunlight.

Finally, regular exercise and physical activities are highly recommended, especially outdoor activities. Exercises and relaxation techniques such as *qi gong* or *tài chí* can also be quite helpful. Inform the patient that inactivity, either physical or mental, is disastrous for most diseases and for general well-being. Mirth, ease, and optimism are factors that should not be underestimated, although their attainment may need some emotional or psychological work. In any case, balanced nutrition, regular exercise, and sunlight are proven factors in emotional and physical well-being.

Endnotes

1   Sun's volume on dietary therapy, translated by Paul Unschuld. Unschuld, P. (1985) *Medicine in China: A History of Ideas*. Berkeley, CA: University of California Press.

2   The latter are taken from the following book and translated: 张湖德, 张玉苹主编. 餐桌上的发物与忌口 [M]. 上海: 上海科学技术出版社. 2007 (Transl.: Zhang Hu-de, Zhang Yu-ping (chief editors): *Fa Wu and Taboos at the Dinner Table* [M]. Shanghai Scientific and Technical Publishers).

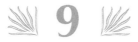

9

Clinical Cases of Psoriasis

IN THE FOLLOWING, a selection of clinical cases will be presented as well as one case series to show how Chinese medicine is applied in practice, and to demonstrate the improvement of psoriasis patients in the course of treatment. Most of the cases were collected during my master's studies at the Dermatology Department of the First Affiliated Hospital of the Zhèjiāng Chinese Medical University, Hángzhōu, China.[1] The time I spent there with Prof. Mǎ Lìlì[2] gave me the opportunity to see a large number of patients with psoriasis of different types and severities over a longer period. All patients had regular appointments at the Dermatology Department so that the course of improvement of psoriasis could be precisely observed and documented.

CLINICAL CASES
#1: Male Patient, 35 Years Old
First Visit

The patient presented at the clinic in October 2013. For more than three years he had been suffering from psoriasis but he had not been cured despite undertaking several therapies. The recurrent skin lesions were found almost all over the body. The lesions always worsened in winter. There was no obvious itching. He had taken some conventional medicine by mail order for more than one year. Initially, the symptoms had subsided. But after stopping the medication, the psoriasis recurred, predominantly on the scalp. He complained about a bitter mouth, dry throat, a quick temper, irritability, yellow urine, and an irregular dry stool (once every 2–3 days).

Specialized skin examination revealed carlet hypertrophic plaques covering the scalp with silver scaling, which ranged from a mungbean-shaped size[3] to a coin-shaped size.[4] This was most severe at the top of the scalp.

Hypertrophic erythema covered with silver scales was seen on the trunk and extremities, with the Auspitz phenomenon (+).

His tongue was red, with a yellow greasy coating and tongue cracks. The pulse was wiry and rapid.

Diagnosis

- TCM: *Bái bǐ*–Liver qì stagnation transforming into Fire syndrome (*gān yù huà huǒ zhèng* 肝郁化火证).

- Western medicine: Psoriasis vulgaris.

Treatment Principle

Clear the Liver, drain fire, and cool the blood (*qīng gān xiè huǒ liáng xuè* 清肝泻火凉血).

Formula

lóng dǎn cǎo	Gentianiae, Radix		6 g
huáng qín	Scutellariae, Radix	*chǎo* (dry fried)	9 g
zhī zǐ	Gardeniae, Fructus	*tàn* (scorched)	9 g
chái hú	Bupleuri, Radix		9 g
dāng guī	Angelicae Sinensis, Radix		9 g
shēng dì huáng	Rehmanniae Glutinosae, Radix		30 g
tōng cǎo	Tetrapanacis, Medulla		6 g
dà huáng	Rhei, Radix et Rhizoma	*chǎo* (dry fried)	5 g
xuán shēn	Scrophulariae Ningpoensis, Radix		9 g
mǔ dān pí	Moutan, Cortex		9 g
chì sháo	Paeoniae Rubrae, Radix		9 g
xià kū cǎo	Spica Prunellae Vulgaris		15 g
gān cǎo	Glycyrrhizae Uralensis, Radix		6 g

Raw herbs taken as a decoction; medication was taken for seven days.

Second Visit

He returned one week later. After the treatment the skin lesions on the scalp, trunk, and extremities were less red and the skin condition had begun to subside. The scales were fewer but still hypertrophic. The bitter mouth and the dry throat had improved. His urine and stools were normal. Due to a lot of work and recent stress, his sleep was lighter and he woke up more easily. His tongue was red, with a thin yellow coating. The pulse was thin and wiry.

Formula Modification

Remove (*chǎo*) *dà huáng* and add *yè jiāo téng* 30 g and (*duàn*) *lóng gǔ* 30 g (boiled first before the other herbs are added) to the last formula (medication for seven days).

Third Visit

The patient returned eight days later. After the treatment the skin lesions had become pale red and the scales were noticeably fewer. His sleep was good, and his urine and stools were normal.

Formula Modification

Remove *yè jiāo téng* and (*duàn*) *lóng gǔ*, while adding *zǐ cǎo* 6 g to the previous formula (medication for 14 days).

Clinical Course

Two weeks later, the skin lesions had subsided by nearly half. The remaining skin lesions were a lot smaller and thinner, pale reddish, and covered by fewer scales.

Discussion

In this case, the patient had had a history of psoriasis for more than three years, accompanied by reddish erythema, which were thick and uplifted as well as covered by many scales. The skin lesions, mainly at the top of the scalp, which is linked to the Liver channel pathway, were hypertrophic, thick, and scarlet. The significance of hypertrophic plaques in this case is remarkable. Remember, "hypertrophic" means well-defined plaques of red, thick, and raised skin lesions due to hyperproliferation of the epidermis, which is a clear sign of psoriasis vulgaris. Along with symptoms including irritability, bitter mouth, dry throat, red tongue with a yellow greasy coating, and a wiry and rapid pulse, this patient was diagnosed with a syndrome of Liver qì stagnation transforming into fire and blood heat transforming into wind exuberance.

The patient was treated with modified *Lóng Dǎn Xiè Gān Tāng*. In this formula, *lóng dǎn cǎo*, (*chǎo*) *huáng qín*, and (*tàn*) *zhī zǐ* were used to clear the Liver and drain Liver fire. To minimize the bitter and cold character of *huáng qín* and *zhī zǐ*, they were dry fried (*chǎo*) and scorched (*tàn*), making them more tolerable for the digestive system. *Chái hú* was used as a Liver channel ushering herb, and as a means to soothe the Liver qì. *Dāng guī* and *shēng dì huáng* were used to nourish Liver blood if too many cold and bitter herbs impaired yīn and blood. *Xuán shēn*, *mǔ dān pí*, *chì sháo*, and *xià kū cǎo* were used to cool the blood and promote blood circulation. *Gān cǎo* was used to harmonize the formula. The whole formula embodied the method of combining "clear heat with drain fire" and "soothe and disperse the Liver" in combination with "nourish and replenish yīn and blood." Thus, Liver fire could be reduced and heat cleared, and blood heat could be diminished in order to cure the skin lesions.

#2: Female Patient, 27 Years Old
First Visit

The patient presented at the clinic in June 2013. Her main complaint was a left-side scalp erythema with itchy scales for more than two months.

History: As a result of an emotional disturbance two months previously, bean-shaped reddish papules, covered by scales, suddenly erupted on the left side of her scalp behind the left ear. This was accompanied by an itching sensation without obvious exudate after scratching. The papules then gradually expanded to coin-shaped skin lesions, which were scarlet, very itchy, and covered by more and thicker silver scales. She also had the Auspitz phenomenon (+). She had a history of lobular hyperplasia of the mammary gland. She complained about sensitivity in her breasts and strain in the lower abdomen during menstruation. Menstrual bleeding was heavy with blood clots.

The tongue was dark red with a greasy thin yellow coating. The pulse was fine and wiry.

Diagnosis

- TCM: *Bái bǐ*–Blood stasis with depressed heat in the Liver channel (*yū xuè nèi zǔ, gān jīng yù rè* 瘀血内阻, 肝经郁热).

- Western medicine: Psoriasis vulgaris.

Treatment Principle

Promote blood circulation, clear the Liver, and drain fire (*huó xuè huà yū jì, qīng gān xiè huǒ* 活血化瘀剂, 清肝泻火).

Formula

lóng dǎn cǎo	Gentianiae, Radix		6 g
huáng qín	Scutellariae, Radix	*chǎo* (dry fried)	9 g
zhī zǐ	Gardeniae, Fructus	*tàn* (scorched)	9 g
chái hú	Bupleuri, Radix		9 g
dāng guī	Angelicae Sinensis, Radix		9 g
shēng dì huáng	Rehmanniae Glutinosae, Radix		30 g
mǔ dān pí	Moutan, Cortex		9 g
chì sháo	Paeoniae Rubrae, Radix		9 g
xuán shēn	Scrophulariae Ningpoensis, Radix		9 g
yì mǔ cǎo	Leonuri, Herba		9 g
líng xiāo huā	Campsis, Flos		9 g
xiāng fù	Cyperi, Rhizoma		9 g
dì fū zǐ	Kochiae Scopariae, Fructus		9 g
dà zǎo	Jujubae, Fructus		9 g
gān cǎo	Glycyrrhizae Uralensis, Radix		6 g

Medication was taken for seven days.

Second Visit

She returned one week later. After treatment, the skin lesions became lighter and less itchy, and there were fewer scales. There was also less tenderness in her breasts. She had recently had a burning sensation during urination and yellow urine. Her stools were normal.

The tongue was dark with a greasy thin yellow coating. The pulse was thin and wiry.

Formula Modification

Add *dàn zhú yè* 9 g and *mù tōng* 6 g to the previous formula (medication for seven days).

Third Visit

The patient came again 11 days later. She said that she had stopped taking the medication for three days because of menstruation. There was no obvious dysmenorrhea and fewer blood clots as well as no distending pain in her breasts. The skin lesions on the left side of the scalp were a lighter red and had far fewer scales. She felt more cheerful this time. Her urine and stools were normal.

The tongue was red with a slight dark, yellow coating. The pulse was fine and wiry.

Formula Modification

Remove *dàn zhú yè* from the last formula (medication for 14 days).

Clinical Course

After one month, the skin lesions on the left side of the scalp had fundamentally subsided with no itching sensation. The distending pain in her breasts during menstruation had gone. There was no dysmenorrhea and no blood clots, and the amount of menstrual blood had increased.

Discussion

In this case, the emotional disturbance had led to Liver depression and qì stagnation. The qì stagnation transformed into fire, which manifested in erythema, papules, and irritability. The heat attacked the skin, which manifested in scales and an itching sensation. The manifestations of this patient indicated the progressive stage of psoriasis and included left-side scalp erythema with thick scales and the Auspitz phenomenon (+). The patient had blood clots in her menstrual blood and showed a dark red tongue, which indicated that there was blood stasis. Therefore, *Lóng Dǎn Xiè Gān Tāng*, plus herbs to promote blood circulation such as *mǔ dān pí, chì sháo*, and *yì mǔ cǎo*, was prescribed in order to promote blood circulation, clear the Liver, and drain fire.

#3: Female Patient, 38 Years Old
First Visit

The patient presented at the clinic in March 2013. Her main complaint was scalp erythema covered by scales, accompanied by an itching sensation for more than six months, aggravated during the previous seven days.

History: Six months ago, for no obvious reason, reddish papules were seen on the front hairline, vertex, and bilateral post-auricular area. The papules were covered by thin silver scales and accompanied by a slight itching sensation. Since that time, the red skin lesions had been gradually growing thicker, expanding into a coin-shaped size and covered by even more scales. After being diagnosed with psoriasis at a local hospital, she was treated with ultraviolet radiation and some correlated therapies, which made the skin lesions subside. Due to a heated argument with her husband seven days previously, red papules on the scalp had returned. They were covered by silver scales and accompanied by a severe itching sensation. Furthermore, she had vertigo, a distending sensation of the head, a dry and bitter mouth, distending pain of the hypochondrium, oppression in the chest and stomach, and insomnia. Her urine was yellow and brown, and she suffered from constipation.

The tongue was red with a yellow greasy coating. The pulse was strong and wiry.

Diagnosis

- TCM: *Bái bǐ*–Depressed heat in the Liver channel (*gān jīng yù rè* 肝经郁热).

- Western medicine: Psoriasis vulgaris.

Treatment Principle

Clear the Liver, drain fire, regulate qì, and relieve depression (*qīng gān xiè huǒ, lǐ qì jiě yù* 清肝泻火, 理气解郁).

Formula

lóng dǎn cǎo	Gentianiae, Radix		6 g
zhī zǐ	Gardeniae, Fructus	*tàn* (scorched)	9 g
huáng qín	Scutellariae, Radix	*chǎo* (dry fried)	9 g
chái hú	Bupleuri, Radix		9 g
huáng lián	Coptidis, Rhizoma		3 g
shēng dì huáng	Rehmanniae Glutinosae, Radix		30 g
xià kū cǎo	Spica Prunellae Vulgaris		12 g
xuán shēn	Scrophulariae Ningpoensis, Radix		9 g
bái jí lí	Tribuli Terristris, Fructus		9 g
bái jú huā	Chrysanthemi, Flos		9 g
zhēn zhū mǔ	Margaritaferae, Concha	(decocted first)	30 g
yè jiāo téng	Polygoni Multiflori, Caulis		30 g
dà huáng	Rhei, Radix et Rhizoma	*chǎo* (dry fried)	5 g
chén pí	Citri Reticulatae, Pericarpium		9 g
gān cǎo	Glycyrrhizae Uralensis, Radix		6 g

Medication taken for seven days.

Directions: Calm the spirit and relax the mind.

Second Visit

She returned eight days later. After the treatment, the skin lesions had become lighter. There were fewer scales and only occasional itching. The symptoms reported at the last visit were much better, but she had recently lost her appetite. Urine and stools were normal.

Her tongue was red with a thin yellow coating. The pulse was fine and wiry.

Formula Modification

Remove *huáng lián* and (*chǎo*) *dà huáng* and add (*chǎo*) *gǔ yá* 9 g, *mài yá* 9 g, and *shān zhā* 6 g to the last formula (medication for seven days).

Third Visit

The patient returned eight days later. The skin lesions had subsided by almost half and there was no obvious itching sensation. She occasionally felt a distending pain in the bilateral post-auricular area. Urine and stools were normal. Appetite and sleep were good. No other signs were reported.

The tongue was pale red with a greasy yellow coating. The pulse was fine and wiry.

Formula Modification

lóng dǎn cǎo	Gentianiae, Radix		6 g
zhī zǐ	Gardeniae, Fructus	*tàn* (scorched)	9 g
huáng qín	Scutellariae, Radix	*chǎo* (dry fried)	9 g
chái hú	Bupleuri, Radix		9 g
shēng dì huáng	Rehmanniae Glutinosae, Radix		30 g
xià kū cǎo	Spica Prunellae Vulgaris		12 g
xuán shēn	Scrophulariae Ningpoensis, Radix		9 g
bái jí lí	Tribuli Terristris, Fructus		9 g
bái jú huā	Chrysanthemi, Flos		9 g
zhēn zhū mǔ	Margaritaferae, Concha	(decocted first)	30 g
fó shǒu	Citri Sarcodactylis, Fructus		9 g
gān cǎo	Glycyrrhizae Uralensis, Radix		6 g

Medication taken for 14 days.

Clinical Course

She came back two weeks later. The scalp skin lesions were cured and she did not report any complaints.

Discussion

Depressed heat in the Liver channel, which is clinically characterized as qì stagnation and constrained heat, belongs to the category of the "Five Depressions" (food, dampness, phlegm, blood, fire) recorded in the Yellow Emperor's Inner Canon, the *Huáng Dì Nèi Jīng*.[5] In this particular case, the patient's manifestations were caused by emotional distress. Liver qì stagnation leads to a disorder of the qì's ascending and descending function, which could transform into fire and push the lucid yáng upwards. Modified *Lóng Dǎn Xiè Gān Tāng* was used to clear the Liver, drain fire, regulate qì, and relieve constraint.

Within this formula, *lóng dǎn cǎo*, *(tàn) zhī zǐ*, and *(chǎo) huáng qín* were used to clear the Liver and drain fire; *shēng dì huáng* was used to nourish yīn and the blood; *xià kū cǎo*, *xuán shēn*, and *huáng lián* were used to clear heat and drain fire; *bái jí lí*, *bái jú huā*, and *zhēn zhū mǔ* were used to clear and calm the Liver as well as subdue yáng; and *fó shǒu* and *chén pí* were used to soothe the Liver and regulate the qì. These herbs were used together to lower Liver fire, regulate qì, and relieve depression in order to cure the skin lesions.

#4: Male Patient, 29 Years Old

As already mentioned, a not inconsiderable number of patients had been taking conventional drugs before they came to us for treatment with TCM. The following case is an excellent example of how TCM can improve the skin appearance and keep it stable. This enabled the patient to reduce and discontinue his conventional medication at a later stage.

First Visit

The patient came into the clinic for the first time in August 2015. One year before, the patient reported, he had had recurrent large and thick red lesions on his left leg. He described the size of the lesions as like mung beans, overlaid with white scales. The lesions were itching slightly and after scratching the rash gradually expanded into a large armor with increased scaling. The rash gradually spread over the trunk and upper limbs. After using topical corticosteroid creams, which he had taken on his own account, the rash had gradually faded. Since then, until May 2015, he had not observed any obvious skin change. But in May 2015, according to the patient, red patches, covered by white scales, had developed on his scalp, both ears, ear canals, armpits, and groin area. The lesions were slightly itchy. Somewhat concerned, he had gone to the local hospital where he was diagnosed with psoriasis for the first time. There, he was treated with an intravenous injection of dexamethasone, which is a systemic glucocorticoid, and a BCG (Bacillus Calmette-Guerin) polysaccharide nucleic acid injection, an immune modulator. He could not remember the exact number of injections, but after receiving the injections the generalized rash had subsided. Unfortunately, the entire rash gradually returned after stopping the intravenous medication. Back home, the patient continued to use topical corticosteroid creams.

During the first visit in August 2015, the patient reported that two weeks previously his torso had had generalized red papules, rice grain to mungbean size, overlain by white scales. Topical corticosteroid creams no longer gave the significant improvement they had done before. Skin examination during the first visit at the clinic clearly showed large coin-shaped bright red skin lesions overlain by thick white scales on the scalp, both ears, ear canals, and nails. The torso showed rice-grain-sized, bright red papules with overlying white scales. Visible on the limbs were multiple, coin-shaped, bright red papules and a rash, partially confluent, with overlying white scales. On the bilateral axillary and inguinal region, thick, hypertrophic deep red plaques covered by white scales could be seen, with the Auspitz phenomenon (+). To summarize, the lesions on the bilateral axillary, inguinal region, and his elbows were the most severe skin lesions, most intense in redness and thickness of the scaling. The skin in general felt very warm.

Further inquiries revealed the following. There was no sore throat, no sleep disturbance, no discomfort, and a normal appetite at that time. The patient affirmed questions about thirst, a dry mouth, and irritability. He also reported a preference for spicy food and alcohol. The physical assessment showed mild edema on the lower extremities, clear consciousness, no fever, and normal body weight; auscultation and percussion showed no abnormal result; and pulse and blood pressure were within the normal range. One week before this examination was conducted, it had been discovered that the stomach biopsy, taken at another hospital, was positive for *Helicobacter pylori*, and lab tests showed that the patient had been suffering from hyperuricemia and hyperlipidemia. The patient reported no history of other major medical diseases such as hepatitis or tuberculosis, and had no food or drug allergies.

The tongue color was red with a thin yellow coating. His pulse was rapid and slippery.

Due to the severity of the manifestation of psoriasis, the patient was admitted to hospital for further treatment and observation.

Diagnosis

- TCM: *Bái bǐ*–Accumulated blood heat (*xuè rè* 血热).

- Western medicine: Psoriasis vulgaris.

Treatment Principle

Cool and invigorate blood, clear heat, and relieve toxicity in order to eliminate lesions (*liáng xuè huó xuè, qīng rè jiě dú xiāo zhǒng* 凉血活血, 清热解毒消肿).

Formula

shuǐ niú jiǎo	Bubali, Cornu	30 g
lóng dǎn cǎo	Gentianiae, Radix	6 g
dāng guī	Angelicae Sinensis, Radix	12 g
chì sháo	Paeoniae Rubrae, Radix	15 g
mǔ dān pí	Moutan, Cortex	12 g
shēng dì huáng	Rehmanniae Glutinosae, Radix	15 g
xuán shēn	Scrophulariae Ningpoensis, Radix	9 g
bái huā shé shé cǎo	Hedyotis Diffusae, Herba	15 g
qī yè yī zhī huā[6]	Paridis, Rhizoma	9 g
lián qiáo	Forsythiae, Fructus	12 g
gān cǎo	Glycyrrhizae Uralensis, Radix	6 g

Due to the severity of the psoriasis, generalized bright red and thick lesions all over the body, and the patient having received several conventional drugs before, the treatment with Chinese herbal medicine was combined with a compound of a glycyrrhizin 120 mg intravenous drip once a day, and a cefuroxime 3 g intravenous drip twice a day, to reduce inflammation and to prevent an infection of the skin. Topical application of calcipotriol and halometasone cream was applied twice daily directly to the psoriasis lesions. Both calcipotriol and halometasone are frequently used in the treatment of psoriasis vulgaris. Calcipotriol is a corticosteroid, an anti-inflammatory agent from the group of vitamin-D3 derivatives, which promotes the formation of normal skin. Halometasone is also a corticosteroid. Halcinonide solution, which is a topical corticosteroid primarily consisting of synthetic steroids, was also applied on the scalp twice a day. It is used as an anti-inflammatory and anti-pruritic agent.

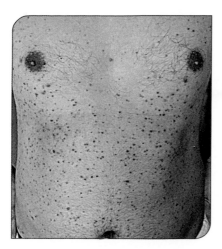
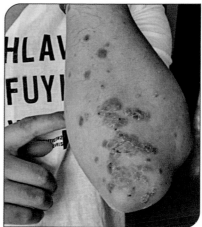
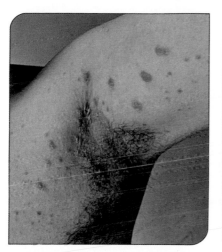
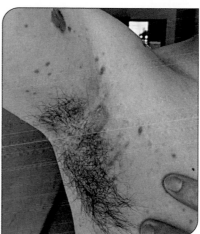
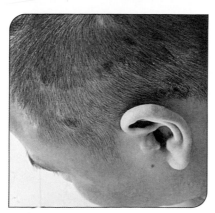
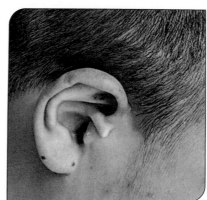

Second Visit

Three days later, the skin lesions on the scalp, trunk, extremities, and in the armpits were visibly less red and thinner, and the scales were fewer. The most obvious changes could be seen on the armpits, inguinal region, and his elbows. These were the areas that had been the most severely affected at the first visit. The skin felt cooler than when he had come in three days before. The patient's tongue and pulse condition were unchanged. The glycyrrhizin and cefuroxime intravenous drips could be reduced and were discontinued some days later. In addition to the internal treatment with Chinese herbal decoctions as described above, external Chinese herbal treatment was added once a day as a wash to clear heat and cool blood.

Formula for External Treatment

kǔ shēn	Sophorae Flavescentis, Radix	15 g
cāng zhú	Atractylodis, Rhizoma	10 g
jīn yín huā	Lonicerae Japonicae, Flos	30 g
bái xiān pí	Dictamni Radicis, Cortex	30 g
shēng dì huáng	Rehmanniae Glutinosae, Radix	20 g
mǎ chǐ xiàn	Portulacae, Herba	30 g
shí liú pí	Granati, Pericarpium	20 g
dì fū zǐ	Kochiae Scopariae, Fructus	30 g

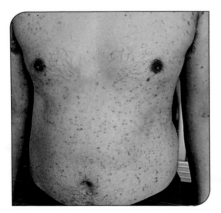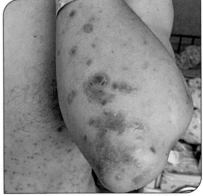

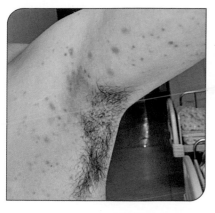
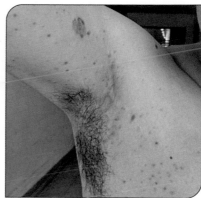
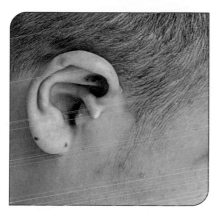
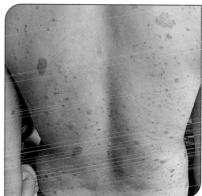

Third Visit

After taking the herbs, his skin had improved significantly. Eleven days later, the skin lesions on the chest and the abdomen had completely disappeared. All other skin lesions had faded and become less red. The scaling had become thinner and was noticeably reduced. The tongue color was less red with a thin yellow coating, and the pulse was less rapid but still slightly slippery. Due to the significant improvement of the appearance of his skin and his good general condition, the patient could be discharged from the hospital later the same day. The topical treatment with conventional drugs (calcipotriol and halometasone cream, plus halcinonide solution) was reduced from twice a day to once a day at discharge. He received a prescription of Chinese herbal medicine for internal and external use for seven days to consolidate his treatment. The patient was instructed to discontinue the conventional topical treatments as soon as all skin lesions disappeared and to come back to the hospital for a follow-up.

Formula for Oral Intake

dāng guī	Angelicae Sinensis, Radix		12 g
mǔ dān pí	Moutan, Cortex		12 g
chì sháo	Paeoniae Rubrae, Radix		15 g
shēng dì huáng	Rehmanniae Glutinosae, Radix		12 g
bái huā shé shé cǎo	Hedyotis Diffusae, Herba		15 g
lián qiáo	Forsythiae, Fructus		12 g
tǔ fú líng	Smilacis Glabrae, Rhizoma		30 g
huò xiāng	Agastachis, Herba		9 g
pèi lán[7]	Eupatorii, Herba		9 g
yì yǐ rén	Coices, Semen	*chǎo* (dry fried)	30 g
zé xiè	Alismatis, Rhizoma		9 g

Medication taken for seven days.

Formula for Fumigation and External Washing

huáng bǎi	Phellodendri, Cortex	30 g
kǔ shēn	Sophorae Flavescentis, Radix	30 g
táo rén	Persicae, Semen	30 g
dì fū zǐ	Kochiae Scopariae, Fructus	30 g
shé chuáng zǐ	Cnidii, Fructus	30 g

Medication taken for seven days.

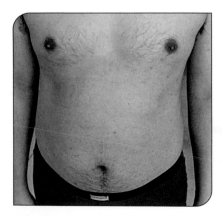
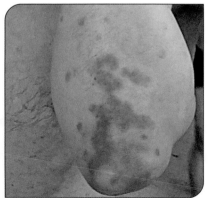

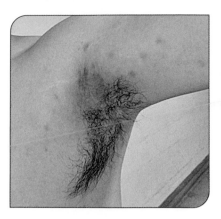
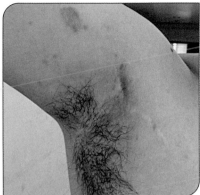
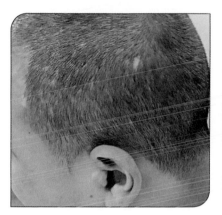
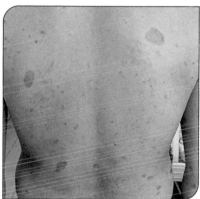

Discussion

This was a particularly severe case of psoriasis vulgaris where hospitalization was required to provide the necessary closely monitored medical care and to observe the patient's further progress. The young male patient's manifestations were caused by the combination of a yáng (heat) constitution and stagnation of pathogenic qì, caused by excessive spicy food and alcohol, and emotional factors. If qì cannot flow freely, it stagnates and accumulates in the body, later on transforming into heat and fire. When extreme heat or fire enters the blood vessels, it sears them, causing an abnormal flow of hot blood. The manifestations on the skin can be seen in the bright red lesions, the very warm skin, and the bleeding of the skin after scratching. It can be often observed that patients feel quite relieved when scratching causes bleeding, as this releases some heat from the blood. With the bright red psoriasis lesions, a red tongue with thin and yellow coating, the rapid and slippery pulse, irritability, dry mouth, and thirst, the patient was diagnosed with the TCM pattern of accumulation of internal blood heat.

An important note at this point: The rapid and slippery pulse at the time of the first visit at the hospital was primarily considered to be a sign of excess heat because heat in the blood belongs to the excess-heat type. According to the pulse condition, the skin appearance, and the other features, a rapid treatment was required and the skin needed more immediate attention. Heat in the blood was a priority in this case. However, if we look at this case from a different angle, the patient most probably also had underlying internal damp-heat. This could be seen from his slippery pulse, which was most likely caused by his improper dietary habits and the drinking of alcohol. Prioritizing damp-heat in the first treatment would not have improved this kind of severe skin condition at that time. As can be seen, damp-heat was taken into account and treated in the final prescription with herbs such as *huò xiāng, pèi lán*, (*chǎo*) *yì yǐ rén*, and *zé xiè*. This approach means a strong and frequently monitored treatment at the beginning to relieve the skin lesions, and a more root-based treatment involving damp-heat clearing at a later stage.

The first formula was a combination of *Xī Jiǎo Dì Huáng Tāng* (Rhinoceros Horn and Rehmannia Decoction) plus some herbs to clear heat, relieve toxicity, and disperse heat. *Qī yè yī zhī huā* is a particularly useful herb to prevent infections and reduce pain on the skin. Dosages of 3–6 g are often enough. In this particularly severe case of psoriasis vulgaris, *qī yè yī zhī huā* was used at a relatively high dosage of 9 g in order to drain heat as effectively as possible, relieve fire toxicity, and reduce swelling and inflammation of the affected skin lesions. The patient received the first formula daily without a break for 14 days. At the third visit, due to the significant improvement of the patient's skin appearance, the formula was changed and adapted to his new situation; in addition, it now addressed the underlying damp condition. The skin looked less red, and the scaling was reduced and noticeably thinner. Herbs such as *shuǐ niú jiǎo, lóng dǎn cǎo*, and *qī yè yī zhī huā* could be removed from the prescription. The treatment with conventional drugs could be reduced and later discontinued, and the topical treatment with conventional drugs could be replaced by external Chinese herbal remedies. The patient was discharged from the hospital in a stable condition with the recommendation for follow-up within a narrow time frame.

In reality, almost all patients who have suffered from psoriasis for a long time have previously received systemic medical treatments with conventional drugs or topical treatment with cortisone. The aim of TCM should always be the reduction of this conventional medication in order to replace it eventually. At the very beginning of a TCM treatment it may be too risky to abruptly discontinue a long-standing therapy with cortisone or other immune-modulatory medications. The body can often not handle these rapid changes and there will be enormous setbacks in the course of the disease. Therefore, it is recommended to gradually reduce the oral and topical treatment with conventional drugs, as can be seen in the case at hand.

Case Series of 56 Patients with Psoriasis on the Head

The key subject of my master's studies in China was psoriasis, particularly scalp psoriasis. My research included investigating the exact mechanisms of this disease and the corresponding treatment options, and to explore the effectiveness and safety of Chinese herbal medicine in the treatment of psoriasis, both using classical TCM and taking into account recent results of biochemical and pharmacological research. As stated previously, the prevalence of psoriasis is increasing, and it seems obvious that this disease has a close relationship to stress. Therefore, my Chinese colleague Fāng Yīmiào and I chose the TCM syndrome of stagnant heat in the Liver channel because this TCM pattern can be frequently observed in patients with psoriasis who have had episodes of severe stress or periods of recurring anger. Since psoriasis often starts on the scalp, we collected data on 56 cases of scalp psoriasis. Based on classical reference material and clinical experience, our hypothesis is that scalp psoriasis is closely related to heat stagnation in the Liver channel, as explained earlier. Targeting the Liver channel, calming the Liver yáng, and clearing Liver heat is therefore supposed to help in the treatment of scalp psoriasis and possibly prevent the spread of psoriasis to other areas of the body. The representative formula for clearing heat stagnation in the Liver channel is *Lóng Dǎn Xiè Gān Tāng*. The usage of bitter-cold herbs such as *lóng dǎn cǎo, huáng qín* and *zhī zǐ* enables a clearing and purging of heat.[8] The following details the course of treatments and the results of our analysis.

Method

Fifty-six patients diagnosed with scalp psoriasis (*tóu bù yín xiè bìng*) with a syndrome of depressed heat in the Liver channel were treated with modified *Lóng Dǎn Xiè Gān Tāng*. The treatment involved one dose taken twice daily, decocted in water for eight consecutive weeks. All patients were evaluated before and after treatment using the Psoriasis Scalp Severity Index (PSSI). Adverse events and data were statistically analyzed. As this was a case series, no ethical approval had to be obtained.

Case Collection, Statistical Methods, Inclusion/Exclusion Criteria, Results
General Data

From January 2013 to August 2014, 56 patients suffering from scalp psoriasis vulgaris were selected and treated at the Dermatology Department of the First Affiliated Hospital of the Zhèjiāng Chinese Medical University, Hángzhōu, China. All patients were chosen in compliance with the TCM Liver meridian syndrome type (see criteria for inclusion in the next section).[9] The 56 patients included 34 males (60.71%) and 22 females (39.29%), aged between 19 and 63 years. The duration of the disease at the first visit was from five months to 30 years. The average duration of the disease in all patients was 6.5 years. There were nine cases of withdrawal (16.1%). The reasons for premature discontinuation of the treatment were lack of efficacy in two subjects (3.6%), the use of topical (external) application in three subjects (5.4%), and non-medical reasons in four subjects (7.1%). At the end of the study, there were 47 patients in total who completed the eight weeks of treatment.

Criteria for Inclusion

1. Diagnostic criteria of scalp psoriasis in the progressive stage: red inflammatory papules on the scalp, rashes and patches of varying sizes, overlying multi-layered silvery white scales, and blood spots under the scales when the skin membrane is ruptured by scratching, known as the Auspitz phenomenon. Hair loss may occur in patches or tufts on the scalp. The erythema can expand beyond the hairline, and lesions can be constantly itchy.

2. Syndrome of heat stagnation in the Liver channel type: scalp lesions bright red, scaly, and itching, with bitter taste in the mouth and dry throat, irritability, and dry stool or yellow urine. Red tongue, with yellow or greasy coating; wiry and/or slippery pulse.

3. Age 18–65 years.

4. Volunteered to participate in this clinical trial and signed the informed consent form.

Exclusion Criteria

1. Age under 18 years or over 65 years.

2. Fungal infections or bacterial infections on the scalp.

3. Suffering from severe seborrheic dermatitis on the scalp and face.

4. Infection, pregnancy, childbirth, trauma, or stress.

5. Systemic or topical application of corticosteroids, immuno-suppressants, and PUVA (psoralen plus UV-A photodynamic therapy) within four weeks before the clinical trial.

6. Severe Heart, Liver, and Kidney disease or mental illness.

Method of Analysis

All patients were treated with modified *Lóng Dǎn Xiè Gān Tāng* for eight consecutive weeks. The herbs were decocted by the Chinese Medicine Preparation Department at the hospital. The medicine was taken twice a day, 200 ml decoction each time. Neither PUVA treatment nor external applications were permitted during the observation period.

Modified *Lóng Dǎn Xiè Gān Tāng* (Gentian Decoction to Drain the Liver):

lóng dǎn cǎo	Gentianiae, Radix		4–6 g
zhī zǐ	Gardeniae, Fructus	*tàn* (scorched)	9 g
chái hú	Bupleuri, Radix		9 g
yù jīn	Curcumae, Radix		9 g
huáng qín	Scutellariae, Radix	*chǎo* (dry fried)	9 g
bái jí lí	Tribuli Terrestris, Fructus		9 g
fú líng	Poriae Cocos, Sclerotium		15 g
bái zhú	Atractylodis Macrocephalae, Rhizoma		9 g
zhēn zhū mǔ	Margaritaferae, Concha	(decocted first)	25 g
zé xiè	Alismatis, Rhizoma		9 g
dà qīng yè	Isatidis, Folium		12 g
shēng dì huáng	Rehmanniae Glutinosae, Radix		15 g

Modifications during the Eight-Week Treatment

For marked erythema, we added *kǔ shēn* 6 g and *shuǐ niú jiǎo* 30 g. For constipation, we added *huái huā* 15 g, (*chǎo*) *dà huáng* 9 g and (*shēng*) *shí gāo*

30 g. For very thick scales, we added *bái xiān pí* 15 g and *yě qiáo mài gēn* 20 g. For hypertrophic plaques, we added *é zhú* 5 g, (*duàn*) *shí jué míng* 30 g and *tǔ fú líng* 15–20 g.

At the first visit, a complete medical history was documented for each patient. A detailed clinical examination, including a routine blood test and a hepatic and renal function test, was performed and was repeated after eight weeks of the treatment. Adverse effects were defined as clinical signs or symptoms that appeared or worsened during the treatment. Patients were seen at the end of two, four, six, and eight weeks. The indicators observed and adverse reactions were checked and recorded. After the eight weeks, all patients were seen on a regular basis for usual skin treatment at the hospital.

Outcome Measures

The grading for the area of scalp lesions: 0 = no lesions; 1 = lesion area < 10%; 2 = lesion area 10–29%; 3 = lesion area 30–49%; 4 = lesion area 50–69%; 5 = lesion area 70–89%; 6 = lesion area > 90%. The indicators for severity of lesions included erythema, scaling, and infiltration. The severity of skin damage: 0 = no lesions; 1 = mild; 2 = moderate; 3 = severe; 4 = severest possible. The Psoriasis Scalp Severity Index (PSSI) = sum of scores for erythema, scaling, and infiltration of the scalp (range 0–72).

Efficacy Criteria

Efficacy was evaluated by the reduced percentage of PSSI severity score shown in Table 1. The efficacy index = [treatment score – points after treatment / treatment score] × 100%. The categories of efficacy were: "full recovery," "very effective," "effective," "ineffective." (Full recovery: efficacy index ≥ 90%; very effective: efficacy index ≥ 60%; effective: efficacy index ≥ 20%; ineffective: efficacy index < 20%.)

Statistical Methods

Application of Statistical Package for Social Sciences (SPSS) 17.0 as statistical software, measurement data represented by (± s), comparing before and after therapy using a paired sample t test; $P < 0.05$ was considered statistically significant. The χ^2 test was used to compare the rates.

Outcome: Evaluation of Efficacy

The PSSI is a commonly used tool for the measurement of the severity of psoriasis. The PSSI score assesses the severity of lesions and the area affected by psoriasis and converts this into a single score in the range from

0 (no disease) to 72 (maximal disease). The PSSI score of our case patients significantly decreased after eight weeks of treatment (see Table 1).

Table 1 PSSI score before and after the treatment of scalp psoriasis lesions

Medication	Cases	Before treatment	After eight weeks of treatment
Modified *LDXGT*	47	19.15 ± 12.85	6.74 ± 5.36

Notes: Compared to before the treatment, t = 8.46, P < 0.001.
± in this table describes the standard deviation of the (mean) PSSI score.
t is the t-statistic: ratio of the average of the difference to the standard error of the difference.
P documents the statistically significant difference.

Table 2 Severity scores before and after treatment of scalp psoriasis lesions with *Lóng Dǎn Xiè Gān Tāng*

Symptoms	Before treatment		After eight weeks of treatment		Percentage of reduction
	Total	Average	Total	Average	
Area	162	3.45 ± 1.52	101	15 ± 1.14	37.65%
Erythema	101	2.15 ± 0.72	53	1.13 ± 0.65	47.52%
Scaling	76	1.62 ± 0.77	44	0.94 ± 0.57	42.11%
Infiltration	64	1.36 ± 0.79	35	0.74 ± 0.68	45.31%
Total score	900	19.15 ± 12.85	317	6.74 ± 5.36	64.78%

Notes: The reduction percentage = [score before treatment − score after treatment] / treatment score × 100%.
One patient's score = Psoriasis Scalp Severity Index (PSSI) = sum of scores for erythema, desquamation,
        and infiltration × involved area (range 0–72).
The total score = the sum of the 47 patients' PSSI score

Table 3 The efficacy of *Lóng Dǎn Xiè Gān Tāng* in the treatment of scalp psoriasis

Medication	Cases	Full recovery	Very effective	Effective	Ineffective	Effective rate
Modified *LDXGT*	47	6	26	10	5	68.1%

Note: Effective rate = [number of cases cured + number of markedly improved cases] / total number of
    cases × 100%.

Adverse Events

No systemic adverse reactions were found in any of the 47 patients who completed the treatment. The routine blood, hepatic, and renal function tests did not show any abnormalities in any of the patients before or after treatment. There were three cases in which adverse reactions occurred locally, the scaling mildly increased in one case, and in one other case a mild stomach pain was observed. These adverse reactions were mild and therefore not a cause to suspend and withdraw from the clinical trial.

Final Conclusion after the Eight Weeks of Treatment with TCM

The clinical data and statistical analysis of the 47 completed cases confirm the feasibility and effectiveness of the modified TCM formula *Lóng Dǎn Xiè Gān Tāng* in the treatment of patients with scalp psoriasis. The PSSI score significantly decreased after the treatment, indicating that Chinese herbal medicine can successfully treat scalp psoriasis caused by the syndrome of heat stagnation in the Liver channel. The most evident improvement was the subsidence of erythema, followed by the improvement of infiltration, degree of scaling, and area size reduction. There were no significant side effects during the treatment and no case of withdrawal from treatment.

The PSSI score after treatment went down from 19.15 ± 12.85 to 6.74 ± 5.36. The difference was significant (P < 0.001). The reduction in erythema (total score for all patients) was 47.52%, infiltration 45.31%, scaling 42.11%, and area size 37.65%. The data we have collected comprised the results of psoriasis patients with a syndrome of depressed heat in the Liver channel. Independent of the TCM syndrome, these results clearly allow us to conclude that TCM as a supplement or as a stand-alone therapy promises a safe and effective treatment, with minimal side effects, and it may be able to prevent lesions from spreading from the head to other areas of the body.

Endnotes

1 Data usage with kind permission of the Zhèjiāng Chinese Medical University, Hángzhōu, China.

2 Mǎ Lìlì: Chief physician at the Dermatology Department of the First Affiliated Hospital of the Zhèjiāng Chinese Medical University, Hángzhōu, China.

3 The size can vary—usually 2–5 mm x 3–4 mm.

4 Round, with a diameter of about 15–25 mm.

5 The work is generally dated by scholars to between the late Warring States period (475–221 BC) and the Hàn Dynasty (206 BC–220 AD).

6 Alternative Chinese names: *zǎo xiū* or *chóng lóu*.

7 *Pèi lán* is available in China, but it is not available everywhere. In some European countries, for instance, it is not available because it contains pyrrolizidine alkaloids (PAs), which can lead to liver carcinomas in long-term use. This is why there are legal limits which restrict the PA value in drugs. In effect, this means that there is no herbal product that fulfills this requirement on the European market.

8 The data in this case series were originally published in the *RCHM Journal* (Register of Chinese Herbal Medicine) (UK), Vol. 12, No. 1, 41–47: "Treatment of scalp psoriasis with modified *Lóng Dǎn Xiè Gān Tāng*–A case series." Data usage with kind permission of the *RCHM Journal*.

9 The study was conducted under the guidance of Prof. Mǎ Lìlì.

Afterword

CHINESE DERMATOLOGY offers a full set of diagnostic and therapeutic principles. Unlike conventional medicine, TCM focuses on herbal therapies oriented towards treating the cause, and not merely procedures suppressing symptoms when treating psoriasis.

Psoriasis is a stubborn and progressive disease, which tends to return after remissions; life-long expenses accompany life-long medical care in the system of conventional medicine. The costs of Western drugs can be crippling–costs that are partly owed to research and approval procedures, but also to the fact that pharmaceutical corporations have become profit-oriented. This is clearly a fact that we should not underestimate: the expense of treatment for either the healthcare system, or each individual patient. Chinese herbal medicine is comparatively affordable. Plus, it is easy in its application for psoriasis patients. The advantage that speaks most for Chinese herbal medicine, though, is its individual approach. The lesson learned is obvious: a single, inflexible approach as so often seen in conventional medicine cannot fit every patient in his or her complexity. Chinese herbal medicine offers this individual, complex, and effective approach.

Appendix I: The External Treatment of Psoriasis with Chinese Medicine

THIS APPENDIX provides a brief outline of external treatment options for psoriasis and describes in detail how to make them. This should be useful to whoever is allowed to make them,[1] but it can also serve as useful background information for patients.

All suggestions mentioned in this appendix should serve as a practical orientation. It is important to take into consideration that different formulas can be used for various TCM patterns. The dosages and compounds can be adjusted; and it should also be taken into account that multiple forms of application can be applied at the same time—a wash first and a cream afterwards, for instance.

Medicinal Baths (*Yào Yù*), Herbal Washes (*Xǐ Dí*), and Wet Compresses (*Shī Fū*)

Baths, washes, and wet compresses are applied to treat persistent lesions with profuse scaling. Herbal washes and wet compresses can be applied once or twice a day for about 15 minutes each time. Medicinal baths should not be taken more than three times a week, and they should not be taken during the acute stage because of the potential risk of secondary inflammation.

A classic example for a medicinal herbal bath:

Yín Xiè Bìng Yù Jì (Psoriasis Bathing Supplement)

kū fán	Alumen Dehydratum	120 g
huā jiāo	Zanthoxyli, Pericarpium	120 g
máng xiāo	Natrii Sulfas	500 g
jú huā	Chrysanthemi, Flos	250 g

This formula is most commonly used for dry and itching lesions with copious scaling. It mainly stops itching, clears heat, and reduces swelling.

Soak the ingredients in 1.5 liters of water for 20–30 minutes. Bring them to a boil, then reduce to a low heat, allowing the herbs to simmer slowly for approximately 30 minutes. Strain the liquid. For application, bathe up to three times per week or apply as a wet compress once or twice a day for about 15 minutes each time on the affected skin lesions. Store the herbal liquid in the fridge, and use a fresh portion for each application, warmed till lukewarm, discarding after use. In general, it is advisable to use the herbs for steaming the affected skin lesions after the cooking process in order to make full use of herbal baths.

Usually, different herbs are combined for external applications for each individual case. The formula depends on the patient's needs: more heat-clearing herbs if the skin is red; more herbs that can relieve itching if the patient complains about strong itching; more herbs that can moisten the skin if the skin is very dry. It might be that one herb suffices for a wash, or that a combination of three or four herbs is required. This and the ratio of the prescribed herbs must be assessed and determined in each case.

A frequently used combination in practice as a wash or as a wet compress is:

jīn yín huā	Lonicerae Japonicae, Flos	15 g
dì fū zǐ	Kochiae Scopariae, Fructus	15 g
cè bǎi yè	Platycladi Cacumen	15 g

The following instructions serve as an example of how to make and apply washes or wet compresses. Herbs can be replaced as required, and dosages can be changed anytime—be flexible. Likewise, more or less water can be used for the boiling process in order to vary the concentration of the medicinal liquid. This example combination contains three herbs. For five herbs, increase the water quantity proportionally. This applies to all external applications described earlier in the book.

Advice for boiling times for external applications in general: Do not boil herbs used in external therapy longer than 30 minutes. As the ingredients should work on the surface, only a light cooking process is required. The standard in practice is a boiling time of approximately 20 minutes. Decoctions taken internally have to work at a deeper level in the body, and therefore they require a longer boiling process in order to reach depth.

Soak the herbs in 500 ml of water for 20–30 minutes. Bring the herbs to a boil and reduce to a low heat, allowing the herbs to simmer slowly for approximately 20 minutes. Strain the liquid. For application, use the liquid as a wash or as a wet compress for at least 15 minutes once or twice a day on the affected skin lesions.

This combination can clear heat, expel dampness, cool blood, relieve itching, and promote healing. It can also be used as a cream at a later stage– that is, when the psoriasis has become chronic and the skin is dark purplish and hard. In this instance, soak the herbs in 300 ml sesame oil for two or three days. Then cook over a gentle heat until the herbs turn dark.[2] Remove the herbal residues, add 100 g beeswax, and melt in the hot oil. Allow the oil to cool, and stir constantly until the texture is thick. Apply the cream once or twice a day on the affected areas of the skin.

Jiě Dú Xǐ Yào (Detoxifying Lotion)

pú gōng yīng	Taraxaci, Herba	30 g
kŭ shēn	Sophorae Flavescentis, Radix	12 g
huáng băi	Phellodendri, Cortex	12 g
lián qiáo	Forsythiae, Fructus	12 g
mù biē zǐ[3]	Momordicae, Semen	12 g
jīn yín huā	Lonicerae Japonicae, Flos	10 g
bái zhǐ	Angelica Dahuricae, Radix	10 g
chì sháo	Paeoniae Rubrae, Radix	10 g
mŭ dān pí	Moutan, Cortex	10 g
gān căo	Glycyrrhizae Uralensis, Radix	10 g

Soak the ingredients in 1.5 liters of water for 20–30 minutes. Bring them to a boil and then reduce to a low heat, allowing the herbs to simmer slowly for approximately 20 minutes. Strain the liquid. While the decoction is still hot, steam the affected part over it. For application, wash the affected area or put a wet compress once or twice a day for about 15 minutes each time on the affected skin lesions. This combination strongly clears heat, resolves toxicity, invigorates the blood, and reduces swelling.

Qīng Rè Jiě Dú Xǐ Jì (Clear Heat and Reduce Toxin Wash)

láng dú[4]	Alocasiae seu Euphorbiae, Radix	10 g
hè shī[5]	Carpesii Abrotanoidis Fructus	10 g
kǔ shēn	Sophorae Flavescentis, Radix	15 g
shé chuáng zǐ	Cnidii, Fructus	15 g
bǎi bù	Stemonae, Radix	15 g
mǎ chǐ xiàn	Portulacae, Herba	15 g
chuān jiāo	Xanthaxyli, Semen	5 g

Soak the ingredients in one liter of water for 20–30 minutes. Bring them to a boil, and then reduce to a low heat, allowing the herbs to simmer slowly for approximately 20 minutes. Strain the liquid. While the decoction is still hot, steam the affected part over it to make full use of the herbal liquid. For application, wash the affected area or put a wet compress once or twice a day for about 15 minutes each time on the affected skin lesions. This combination strongly clears heat, resolves fire toxicity, dries dampness, and cools the blood.[6]

Sān Huáng Xǐ Jì (The Yellow Cleanser Formula)

dà huáng	Rhei, Radix et Rhizoma	10 g
huáng bǎi	Phellodendri, Cortex	10 g
huáng qín	Scutellariae, Radix	10 g
kǔ shēn	Sophorae Flavescentis, Radix	10 g

See the instructions for the previous formula for the boiling process. The amount of water for boiling here is 500 ml. For application, wash the affected area or apply a wet compress once or twice a day for about 15 minutes each time. Sān Huáng Xǐ Jì can also be applied with a cotton ball dipped into it, up to three times a day. It clears heat, relieves inflammation, arrests secretion, and stops itching.

Frequently Used Herbs for Medicinal Baths, Cold Wet Compresses, and Herbal Washes

Frequently used herbs for medicinal baths and cold wet compresses in external psoriasis treatment are: mǎ chǐ xiàn, kǔ shēn, huáng bǎi, dì fū zǐ, and *bái xiān pí*. Herbs are chosen according to their action to clear heat, eliminate dampness, reduce swelling, and ease itching.

Frequently used herbs for herbal washes are: *jú huā* or *yě jú huā*, *jīn yín huā*, *pú gōng yīng*, *dì fū zǐ*, *kǔ shēn*, *cè bǎi yè*, *ài yè*, and *qín pí*. Herbal washes with these herbs are most suitable for clearing heat and eliminating itching and dampness. Furthermore, herbs such as *dì fū zǐ*, *kǔ shēn*, *cè bǎi yè*, *ài yè*, and *qín pí* are known to have a skin-moisturizing effect and they can reduce scaling.

It needs to be mentioned here that one should inform the patient that the decocted herbs for external washing should always be kept in the refrigerator; the same applies for herbs you prescribe your patients for oral intake. This will keep them fresh and aromatic. Be careful to avoid contaminating the liquid when taking out portions for use; otherwise, the stock liquid becomes dirty and can contaminate the lesions. After six or seven days, the liquid should no longer be used, because it is not aromatic and fresh anymore, and therefore no longer effective.

For practical reasons, it can also be helpful to inform the patient that some herbs leave stains, such as *huáng bǎi* or *huáng lián*. They should not use white towels and should avoid wearing light-colored clothing while using those medicinals. If patients are advised to do a hand bath, it can be helpful if they have the bath in the evening or at times where they do not have to go to work, because of the staining effect. The yellowish or dirty color can be quite annoying, and if these herbs absolutely must be used, one should carefully explain this to the patient.

Ointments (*Yóu Gāo*, Oil-based Ointments) ▬▬▬

Frequently used herbs for the preparation of oil-based ointments in the case of blood-heat patterns are, for example, *qīng dài* used in *Qīng Dài (Yóu) Gāo* or *huáng lián* used in *Huáng Lián Gāo*.[7]

Qīng Dài (Yóu) Gāo (Indigo Naturalis Ointment)

qīng dài	Indigo Naturalis	60 g
huáng bǎi	Phellodendri, Cortex	60 g
huá shí	Talcum	120 g
shí gāo	Gypsum Fibrosum	120 g

The ingredients mentioned above are *Qīng Dài Sǎn* (Indigo Powder), a popular formula with widely used variations to treat skin conditions. For application, grind the ingredients (except *qīng dài*) to a fine powder and soak them in 500 ml of sesame oil for 24 hours. Cook over a gentle heat until the ingredients have a dark yellow color. Filter off the sesame oil and add *qīng dài* to the medicated oil and mix well. Allow to gel and apply once or twice a day on the affected areas of the skin.

Huáng Lián Gāo (Coptidis Balm)

huáng qín	Scutellariae, Radix	12 g
huáng lián	Coptidis, Rhizoma	10 g
jiāng huáng	Curcumae Longae, Rhizoma	10 g
dāng guī	Angelicae Sinensis, Radix	15 g
shēng dì huáng	Rehmanniae Glutinosae, Radix	15 g

For application, grind the ingredients to a fine powder and soak them in 500 ml of sesame oil for 24 hours. Cook over a gentle heat until the ingredients have a dark yellow color. Filter off the sesame oil, allow to gel, and apply the ointment once or twice a day on the affected areas of the skin.

Both ointments perform a strong action in clearing heat, dispelling toxins, relieving inflammation, and stopping any itching. In clinical experience, herbs such as *qīng dài* or *huáng lián* seem to have very strong effects and can be used as stand-alone herbs in ointments. You do not need to add all herbs mentioned to reach the desired effect. It should be mentioned, however, that these kinds of ointments should only be prescribed when there is no suppuration and skin fissures are closed.

Other commonly used examples of ointments are:

Qīng Liǎn Gāo (Clearing and Cooling Ointment)[8]

dāng guī	Angelicae Sinensis, Radix	30 g
zǐ cǎo	Arnebiae seu Lithospermi, Radix	6–10 g

Qīng Liǎn Gāo nourishes, moistens, and invigorates the blood while clearing heat. It is an ideal choice in the treatment of psoriasis caused by blood heat, blood stasis, or blood deficiency with dryness. For application, soak *dāng guī* and *zǐ cǎo* in 300 ml of sesame oil for two or three days. Then cook over a gentle heat until the herbs turn a dark yellow. Remove the herbal residues and allow the oil to cool before applying to the skin. Apply the ointment once or twice a day on the affected areas of the skin.

This ointment is also known as *Rùn Jī Gāo* (Flesh-Moistening Ointment)[9] when, in addition to *zhī má yóu* (sesame oil), it is mixed with 90–120 g *fēng là* (beeswax). The texture is somewhat thicker, but the effect remains the same: moisturizing the skin, clearing heat from the blood, and alleviating any itching. When *zǐ cǎo* is not available, use the first two formulas (*Qīng Dài Gāo* and *Huáng Lián Gāo*).

Pǔ Lián Gāo (Universally Linked Ointment), also called *Qín Bǎi Gāo* (*Qín Bǎi* Cream)

| *huáng qín* | Scutellariae, Radix | 10 g |
| *huáng bǎi* | Phellodendri, Cortex | 10 g |

Pǔ Lián Gāo clears heat, reduces swelling, moisturizes the skin, and stops itching. For application, grind the herbs into a fine powder and soak them in 250 ml of sesame oil for 24 hours. Cook over a gentle heat until the ingredients have a dark yellow color. Finally, filter off the sesame oil and allow to gel. Apply the ointment once or twice a day on the affected skin lesions.

Yù Huáng Gāo (Jade Yellow Plaster)

dāng guī	Angelicae Sinensis, Radix	30 g
bái zhǐ	Angelica Dahuricae, Radix	9 g
gān cǎo	Glycyrrhizae Uralensis, Radix	30 g
jiāng huáng	Curcumae Longae, Rhizoma	9 g
qīng fěn[10]	Calomelas	6 g
bīng piàn	Borneolum	3 g

Grind the herbs into a fine powder and mix them well with 300 ml of sesame oil. Soak for about 24 hours. The next day, bring the mixture to a boil over a gentle heat, filter off the sesame oil, and allow to gel. Remove the herbal residues and allow the oil to cool. Mix it with beeswax before applying on the skin. Note that in winter usually less beeswax is used than in summer. Apply the ointment once or twice a day on the affected areas of the skin. It clears heat, resolves toxicity, invigorates the blood, and breaks up blood stasis; it reduces swelling and alleviates pain. It is most suitable in blood heat and toxic heat with blood stagnation. Like most other combinations, this can also be used as a wash.

Liú Huáng Gāo (Sulfur Ointment)

liú huáng	Sulfur	5–10 g

Sulfur ointment is another option if there are very thick lesions with serious scaling, pain, and swelling. It clears heat, reduces toxicity, invigorates blood, and stops itching. As it can relieve inflammation, it is often given in the case of bacterial super-infection. For application, grind *liú huáng* into a fine powder and mix it well with 90–95 ml of sesame oil. Bring it to a boil over a gentle heat, filter off the sesame oil, and allow to gel. Apply once or twice a day on the skin lesions. Sulfur ointment is very effective, but the color and the smell has to be considered, and patients must be informed about these downsides before use.

This prescription is also known as *Liú Huáng Ruǎn Gāo*[11] (Sulfur Ointment) when, instead of sesame oil, it is mixed with about 90–95 g beeswax. The texture is somewhat thicker as in *Liú Huáng Gāo*, but the effect remains the same. However, one can add a tiny amount of sesame oil (or jojoba oil) to make the consistency more spreadable.

Zǐ Cǎo Yóu (Self-Made *Zǐ Cǎo* Ointment)

Grind *zǐ cǎo* (approximately 15 g) into a fine powder and mix it well with 100 ml of sesame oil. Soak for three or four days. *Zǐ cǎo* then becomes soft and has to be boiled only for a very short time over a gentle heat. Remove the herbal residues as usual and allow the oil to cool. It can be mixed with beeswax or creams before applying on the skin. It can also be used without the boiling process if *zǐ cǎo* has become soft enough to almost dissolve. Apply the ointment once or twice a day on the affected areas of the skin. *Zǐ cǎo* is strong enough to use as a stand-alone herb in patients with blood heat. It can also be used as a wash.

Diān Dǎo Sǎn Gāo (Upside Down Powder Paste)

| dà huáng | Rhei, Radix et Rhizoma | 10 g |
| liú huáng | Sulfur | 10 g |

Grind the herbs into a fine powder[12] and mix them well with 250 ml sesame oil. Soak for about 24 hours. The next day, bring to a boil over a gentle heat, filter off the sesame oil, and allow to gel. Remove the herbal residues and allow the oil to cool. It can be mixed with beeswax before applying on the skin, but this is not essential. Apply the ointment once or twice a day on the affected areas of the skin. It clears heat and cools the blood. This combination can be used as a wash as well.

It is important to mention at this point that there is a big difference in effectiveness when the herbs are ground (pulverized). The process of grinding enlarges the surface, enabling much more substance to enter the decoction during the soaking and cooking process. In practice, we have found that oil-based lotions that have not been ground or pulverized are not as powerful and effective.

Creams (Rǔ Gāo)

All the ointments mentioned above can also be prepared as creams. These creams have a more solid texture, as the sesame oil is replaced with the natural thickeners of beeswax, cocoa butter, or shea butter. Creams are more appropriate for application to exposed skin areas such as the face and hands. The proportions can be varied depending on individual needs; there are no strict specifications regarding ratios.

For psoriasis, qīng dài cream with or without additions is frequently prescribed and we have had very good clinical experience with it. An advantage of creams is their better retention on the skin. An important consideration is that patients have to feel comfortable with the texture and dark color of qīng dài cream. Advise patients therefore to use dark creams at night, and also not to wear light-colored clothing because the creams will stain.

Qīng Dài Gāo (Indigo Cream)

| Qīng Dài Sǎn | Indigo Naturalis Powder | 75 g |

Melt natural white beeswax over a low heat and allow it to cool. Then add finely powdered *qīng dài* to the beeswax in a proportion of 1:4 and mix well. For a more fluid and smoother consistency, add a tiny amount of sesame oil or jojoba oil to make the cream more spreadable.

Qīng dài can clear heat, resolve toxicity, cool blood, reduce swelling, and inhibit the growth of cells. Thus, *qīng dài* cream is suitable in patterns of blood heat, Liver heat, *yíng*-level heat, or heat-toxin.

When it comes to creams, again it is important to refrain from using Vaseline. Vaseline, as a by-product of the oil industry, is not a high-quality solution. The use of natural ingredients as carrier substances in our products should always be preferred.

Finally, a general note on the application and handling of creams. It is not recommended to rub the whole lesion with cream, as this may enlarge the lesion. This applies to all skin diseases, not just psoriasis. One applies cream from the middle to just before the edge of the affected skin lesion. The cream then penetrates by itself to the surrounding skin. In psoriasis, the skin on the affected area later falls off.

Here is an illustration[13] for clarification:

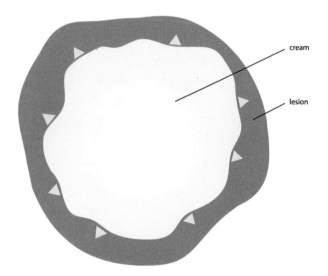

cream

lesion

Tinctures (*Dīng Jì*)

Tinctures, herbal preparations made in alcoholic bases, are not as commonly used in the treatment of psoriasis compared with washes, ointments, and creams. The alcohol that is most often used as a solvent is high-proof alcohol (at least 75%). Generally, the ratio of dried herbs to alcohol is 1:4 or 1:5, and the soaking time of tinctures is about 10–14 days, but there will always be exceptions to this. Tinctures are applied topically on the affected area of the skin. It is important to check the skin before application, because tinctures should not be applied on injured skin areas.

Bǔ Gǔ Zhī Dīng (Bǔ Gǔ Zhī Tincture)

One example of a self-made tincture for external use is bǔ gǔ zhī tincture (bǔ gǔ zhī dīng), as previously mentioned. The average ratio of dried herbs to alcohol is 1:4 or 1:5 and the soaking time is at least ten days. Another example of a tincture is the following combination: xuè jié 5 g, liǔ suān[14] 5 g, and zhāng nǎo 2 g. This combination can clear heat, relieve toxicity, invigorate the blood, and alleviate pain. Powder and mix all components with bì má yóu (castor oil) 10 g and let it soak for 24 hours. Add to 100 ml 90% alcohol and mix well. Generally, the soaking time of tinctures is at least ten days before straining the tincture through a fine sieve into a dark glass. In this particular case, one can use the tincture immediately. Apply once a day on the affected area of the skin. Store the tincture in a cool, dark place. High-proof alcohol acts as a preservative, and if stored properly in a cool dark place, tinctures can have a shelf life of 7–10 years. Again, the use of tinctures in psoriasis is very rarely seen in practice.

Endnotes

1   In some European countries, clinicians are not allowed to make external applications such as creams. This is done by official pharmacies.

2   This process can be very fast. Ten minutes can often be enough, so be careful and observe the cooking process. Otherwise, the oil turns too dark and the smell is too strong.

3   If available.

4   If available.

5   If available.

6   This combination is also useful to expel parasites.

7   From Yī Zōng Jīn Jiàn (The Golden Mirror of Ancestral Medicine).

8   Prof. Zhào Bǐng Nán's clinical experience. Some books mention dà huáng as an additional ingredient, e.g. Xú Xiàngcái, Complete External Therapies of Chinese Drugs, Foreign Languages Press (January 1, 1998).

9   From Wài Kē Zhèng Zōng (True Lineage of External Medicine, 1617).

10 If available.

11 Liú Huáng Gāo 硫磺膏; Liú Huáng Ruǎn Gāo 硫磺软膏.

12 This is called Diān Dǎo Sàn (Upside Down Powder).

13 Illustration by Sabine Schmitz © 2018.

14 Alternative name for liǔ suān (salicylic acid): shuǐ yáng suān.

Appendix II: Colored Tongue Atlas

THIS APPENDIX ILLUSTRATES the different tongues seen in individual TCM patterns. It should be mentioned that in clinical practice patterns often overlap, and therefore clear forms of tongues are not always seen. Each tongue image is briefly described to illustrate the different patterns.

Heat Stagnation in the Liver Meridian
(*Gān Jīng Yù Rè* 肝经郁热)

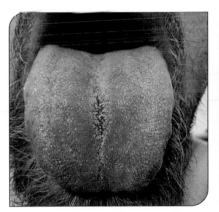

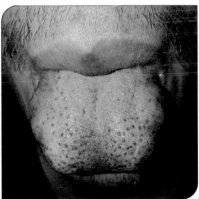

A red tongue with a yellow coating and a crack in the middle. This indicates more heat than dampness and a deficiency of the middle *jiāo*.

The tongue is red with a yellow coating, which indicates internal heat and dampness.

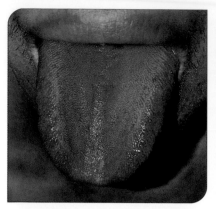

The tongue is red with a very thin yellow coating, which indicates internal heat and mild dampness.

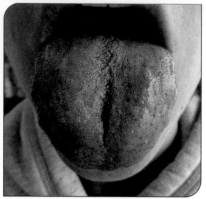

The tongue is red with a yellow coating, which indicates internal heat and some dampness.

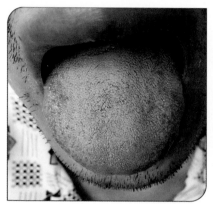

The tongue is red, especially at the borders, which correspond to the Liver in Chinese medicine. The tongue coating is thin and yellow.

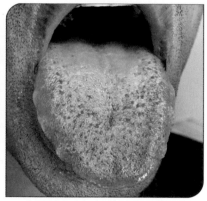

The tongue is red, which indicates internal heat. The tongue coating is thick and yellow.

Accumulated Blood Heat (*Xuè Rè* 血热)

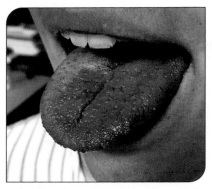

A bright red tongue with prickles, which indicates the consumption of body fluids.

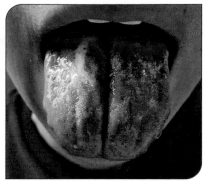

A very red tongue with prickles.

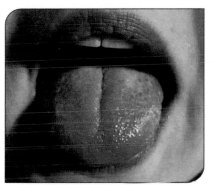

A very red tongue with a thin yellow coating.

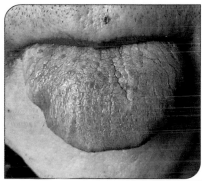

Blood heat turning into stasis and consuming yīn (blood).

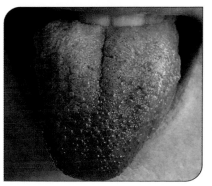

The tongue is scarlet and dry with obvious prickles and a little coating.

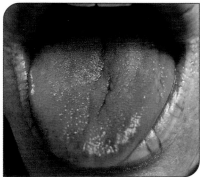

A very red tongue with little coating.

Wind-Heat (*Fēng Rè* 风热)

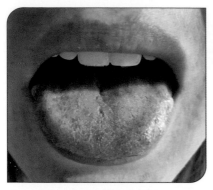

A tongue with a red tip and thin coating.

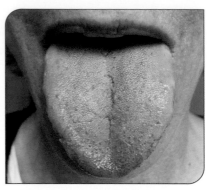

A tongue with a red tip and thin coating.

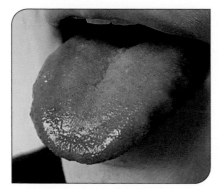

A tongue with a red tip.

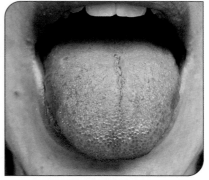

A tongue with a thin yellow coating and a red tip with red spots.

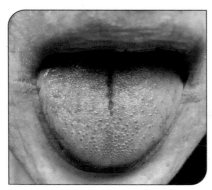

A tongue with red spots on the tip of the tongue and a thin coating.

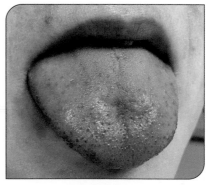

When wind combines with heat, the tip of the tongue is particularly red.

Blood Deficiency and Wind Dryness
(*Xuè Xū Fēng Zào* 血虚风燥)

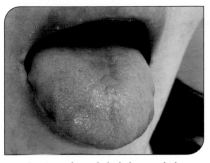

A very pale and slightly purplish tongue with purplish lips, which indicates stagnant blood. If there is not enough blood, it tends to stagnate.

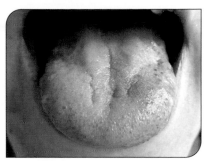

Blood and qì deficiency. The tongue is pale and soft, with tooth-marked tongue borders.

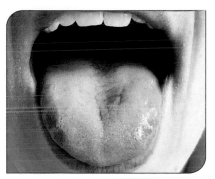

A pale tongue with tooth-marks. This indicates blood deficiency combined with weakness of Spleen qì, which, as a result, is unable to produce blood.

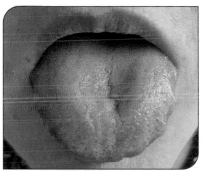

Qì and blood deficiency. A pale, puffy, and tooth-marked tongue body.

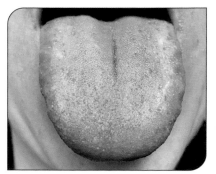

Blood deficiency with some blood stasis. The tongue is pale and slightly purplish.

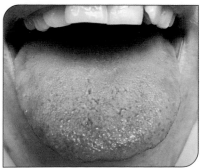

A pale tongue with a thin white coating.

Blood Stagnation (*Xuè Yū* 血瘀)

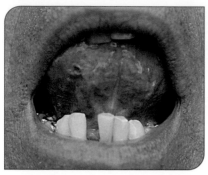

A livid (purple or dark) tongue with purplish veins underneath the tongue.

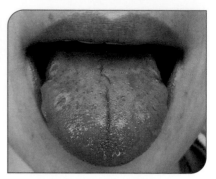

Blood stasis with dampness. A purplish, thick tongue with a white coating at the root.

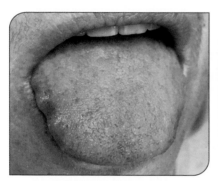

A pale and purplish tongue, which indicates stagnant blood. A tooth-marked tongue body, which indicates qì deficiency.

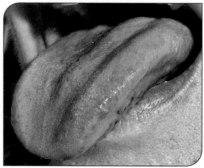

A pale and slightly purplish tongue with stasis spots underneath the tongue.

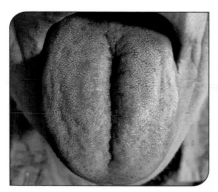

A purplish and puffy tongue with a thin white coating.

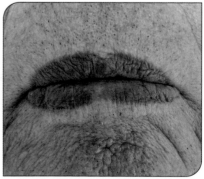

Purplish lips with stasis spots.

Qì Deficiency (*Qì Xū* 气虚)

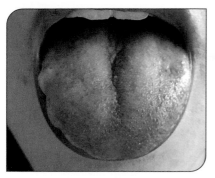

A puffy and pale red tongue with a thin coating and tooth-marks.

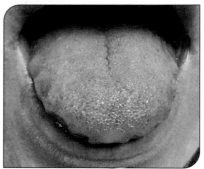

A puffy and tooth-marked tongue. Purplish, thick tongue with a white coating at the root.

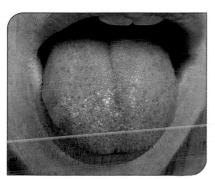

A puffy tongue, pale red.

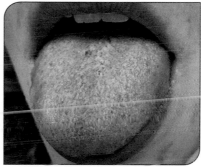

A puffy tongue with tooth-marks and a thick white tongue coating, which indicates qì deficiency with retention of dampness.

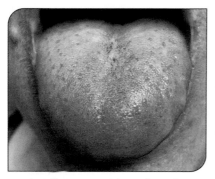

A puffy tongue with tooth-marks and a white coating, which indicates retention of dampness within the body.

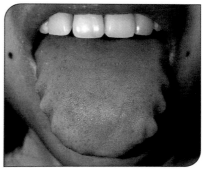

A puffy tongue with tooth-marks.

Dampness-Heat (*Shī Rè* 湿热)

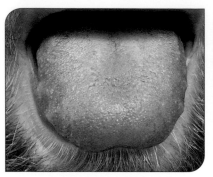

A puffy and red tongue with
a thick yellow coating.

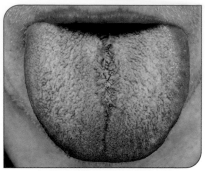

A red tongue with a thick and
greasy yellow coating due to
stress, alcohol, and smoking.

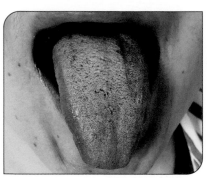

A red tongue with a thick yellow coating.

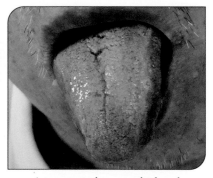

A tongue with a very thick and
greasy yellow coating.

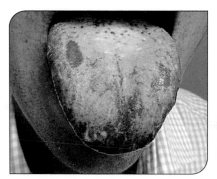

A tongue with a thick yellow and
greasy coating that is peeling in
some places, which can be a sign of
the beginning of yīn deficiency.

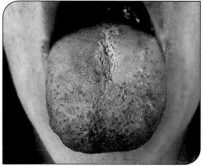

A slightly red tongue with a
thick yellow coating.

Appendix III: *Pīnyīn*–
Chinese–English Formula
Cross-Reference

Pīnyīn	Chinese	English
Bái Hǔ Tāng	白虎汤	White Tiger Decoction
Bì Xiè Shèn Shī Tāng	萆薢渗湿汤	Dioscorea Decoction to Leach Out Dampness
Bǔ Gǔ Zhī Dīng	补骨脂酊	*Bǔ Gǔ Zhī* Tincture
Dān Zhī Xiāo Yáo Sǎn	丹栀逍遥散	Moutan and Gardenia Rambling Powder
Diān Dǎo Sǎn Gāo	颠倒散膏	Upside Down Powder Paste
Èr Miào Sǎn	二妙散	Mysterious Wonder Powder
Fáng Fēng Tōng Shèng Wán	防风通圣丸	Ledebouriella Powder That Sagely Unblocks
Huáng Lián Gāo	黄连膏	Coptidis Balm
Huáng Lián Jiě Dú Tāng	黄连解毒汤	Coptis Decoction to Relieve Toxicity
Jiě Dú Xǐ Yào	解毒洗药	Detoxifying Lotion
Jīn Huáng Sǎn	金黄散	Golden Yellow Powder
Liú Huáng Gāo	硫磺膏	Sulfur Ointment
Liú Huáng Ruǎn Gāo	硫磺软膏	Sulfur Ointment
Liù Jūn Zǐ Tāng	六君子汤	Six Gentlemen Decoction
Lóng Dǎn Xiè Gān Tāng	龙胆泻肝汤	Gentian Decoction to Drain the Liver
Pǔ Lián Gāo	普联膏	Universally Linked Ointment
Qín Bǎi Gāo	芩柏膏	*Qín Bǎi* Cream
Qīng Dài Gāo	青黛膏	Indigo Naturalis Ointment
Qīng Dài Sǎn	青黛散	Indigo Powder
Qīng Liǎn Gāo	清脸膏	Clearing and Cooling Ointment
Qīng Rè Jiě Dú Xǐ Jì	清热解毒洗剂	Clear Heat and Reduce Toxin Wash

Pīnyīn	Chinese	English
Qīng Wēn Bài Dú Yǐn	清瘟败毒饮	Clear Epidemics and Overcome Toxin Decoction
Qīng Yíng Tāng	清营汤	Clear the Nutritive Level Decoction
Rùn Jī Gāo	润肌膏	Flesh-Moistening Ointment
Sān Huáng Xǐ Jì	三黄洗剂	Three Yellow Cleanser Formula
Sháo Yào Dì Huáng Tāng	芍药地黄汤	*Sháo Yào Dì Huáng* Decoction
Sì Jūn Zǐ Tāng	四君子汤	Four Gentlemen Decoction
Sì Wù Tāng	四物汤	Four Substance Decoction
Sōu Fēng Shùn Qì Wán	搜风顺气丸	Track Down Wind and Smooth the Flow of Qi Pill
Táo Hóng Sì Wù Tāng	桃红四物汤	Four Substance Decoction with Safflower and Peach Kernel
Xī Jiǎo Dì Huáng Tāng	犀角地黄汤	Rhinoceros Horn and Rehmannia Decoction
Yín Qiào Sǎn	银翘散	Honeysuckle and Forsythia Powder
Yín Xiè Bìng Yù Jì	银屑病浴剂	Psoriasis Bathing Supplement
Yù Huáng Gāo	玉黄膏	Jade Yellow Plaster
Zēng Yè Tāng	增液汤	Increase the Fluids Decoction
Zǐ Cǎo Yóu	紫草油	Self-Made *Zǐ Cǎo* Ointment

Appendix IV: *Pīnyīn*–Chinese–English Herb Cross-Reference

Pīnyīn	Chinese	Pharmaceutical
ài yè	艾叶	Artemisiae Argyi, Folium
bǎi bù	百部	Stemonae, Radix
bǎi hé	百合	Lilii, Bulbus
bái huā shé shé cǎo	百花蛇舌草	Hedyotis Diffusae, Herba
bái jí lí	白蒺藜	Tribuli Terristris, Fructus
bái máo gēn	白茅根	Imperatae, Rhizoma
bái sháo	白芍	Paeonia Albiflora, Radix
bái xiān pí	白鲜皮	Dictamni Radicis, Cortex
bái zhǐ	白芷	Angelica Dahuricae, Radix
bái zhú	白术	Atractylodis Macrocephalae, Rhizoma
ban lán gēn	板蓝根	Isatidis, Radix
bàn xià	半夏	Pinelliae, Rhizoma
bàn zhī lián	半枝莲	Scutellariae Barbatae, Radix
bì má yóu	蓖麻油	Castor Oil
bì xiè	萆薢	Dioscoreae, Rhizoma
bīng piàn	冰片	Borneolum
bò hé	薄荷	Menthae, Herba
bǔ gǔ zhī	补骨脂	Psoraleae, Fructus
cāng zhú	苍术	Atractylodis, Rhizoma
cè bǎi yè	侧柏叶	Platycladi Cacumen
chái hú	柴胡	Bupleuri, Radix
chē qián zǐ	车前子	Plantaginis, Semen
chén pí	陈皮	Citri Reticulatae, Pericarpium
chì sháo	赤芍	Paeoniae Rubrae, Radix
chóng lóu	重楼	Paridis, Rhizoma

Pīnyīn	Chinese	Pharmaceutical
chuān jiāo	川椒	Xanthaxyli, Semen
chuān niú xī	川牛膝	Cyathulae, Radix
chuān xiōng	川芎	Chuanxiong, Rhizoma
dà huáng	大黄	Rhei, Radix et Rhizoma
dà qīng yè	大青叶	Isatidis, Folium
dà zǎo	大枣	Jujubae, Fructus
dài dài huā	代代花	Citri Aurantii Amarae, Flos
dàn dòu chǐ	淡豆豉	Sojae Praeparata, Semen
dān shēn	丹参	Salviae Miltiorhizae, Radix
dàn zhú yè	淡竹叶	Lophatheri, Herba
dāng guī	当归	Angelicae Sinensis, Radix
dǎng shēn	党参	Codonopsis, Radix
dì fū zǐ	地肤子	Kochiae Scopariae, Fructus
dì gǔ pí	地骨皮	Lycii, Cortex
dú huó	独活	Angelicae Pubescentis, Radix
ē jiāo	阿胶	Asini Corii, Colla
é zhú	莪术	Curcumae, Rhizoma
fáng fēng	防风	Saposhnikoviae, Radix
fēng fáng	蜂房	Vespae, Nidus (Wasp Nest)
fēng là	蜂蜡	Cera Flava
fó shǒu	佛手	Citri Sarcodactylis, Fructus
fú líng	茯苓	Poriae Cocos, Sclerotium
fú píng	浮萍	Spirodelae, Herba
gān cǎo	甘草	Glycyrrhizae Uralensis, Radix
gé gēn	葛根	Puerariae, Radix
gǒu qǐ zǐ	枸杞子	Lycii, Fructus
gǔ yá	谷芽	Oryzae Germinatus, Fructus
hàn lián cǎo	旱莲草	Ecliptae, Herba
hé huān huā	合欢花	Albiziae, Flos
hè shī	鹤虱	Carpesii Abrotanoidis Fructus
hé shǒu wū	何首乌	Polygoni Multiflori, Radix
hóng huā	红花	Carthami, Flos
huā jiāo	花椒	Zanthoxyli, Pericarpium
huá shí	滑石	Talcum
huái huā	槐花	Sophorae Immaturus, Flos

Pīnyīn	Chinese	Pharmaceutical
huái niú xī	怀牛膝	Achyranthis Bidentatae, Radix
huáng bǎi	黄柏	Phellodendri, Cortex
huáng lián	黄连	Coptidis, Rhizoma
huáng qí	黄芪	Astragali, Radix
huáng qín	黄芩	Scutellariae, Radix
huǒ má rén	火麻仁	Cannabis, Semen
huò xiāng	藿香	Agastachis, Herba
jī xuè téng	鸡血藤	Spatholobi, Caulis
jiāng huáng	姜黄	Curcumae Longae, Rhizoma
jié gěng	桔梗	Platycodi, Radix
jīn yín huā	金银花	Lonicerae Japonicae, Flos
jīng jiè	荆芥	Schizonepetae, Herba
jú huā	菊花	Chrysanthemi, Flos
jú yè	橘叶	Citri Reticulatae, Folium
kū fán	枯矾	Alumen Dehydratum
kǔ shēn	苦参	Sophorae Flavescentis, Radix
láng dú	狼毒	Alocasiae seu Euphorbiae, Radix
lián qiáo	连翘	Forsythiae, Fructus
líng xiao huā	凌霄花	Campsis, Flos
liú huáng	硫磺	Sulfur
liǔ suān	柳酸	Salicylic Acid
lóng dǎn cǎo	龙胆草	Gentianiae, Radix
lóng gǔ	龙骨	Calcinated Draconis, Os
lǜ è méi	绿萼梅	Armeniacae Mume, Flos
lú gēn	芦根	Phragmitis, Rhizoma
mǎ chǐ xiàn	马齿苋	Portulacae, Herba
mài mén dōng	麦门冬	Ophiopogonis Japonici, Tuber
mài yá	麦芽	Hordei Germantus, Fructus
máng xiāo	芒硝	Natrii Sulfas
méi guī huā	玫瑰花	Rosae Rugosae, Flos
mù biē zǐ	木鳖子	Momordicae, Semen
mǔ dān pí	牡丹皮	Moutan, Cortex
mù guā	木瓜	Cydonium Sineuse
mù hú dié	木蝴蝶	Oroxylum, Semen
mù tōng	木通	Akebiae, Caulis

Pīnyīn	Chinese	Pharmaceutical
niú bàng zǐ	牛蒡子	Arctii Lappae, Fructus
niú xī	牛膝	Achyranthis, Radix
pèi lán	佩兰	Eupatorii, Herba
pú gōng yīng	蒲公英	Taraxaci, Herba
qī yè yī zhī huā	七叶一枝花	Paridis, Rhizoma
qiāng huó	羌活	Notopterygii, Rhizoma Seu Radix
qín pí	秦皮	Fraxini, Cortex
qīng dài	青黛	Indigo Naturalis
qīng fěn	轻粉	Calomelas
quán xiē	全蝎	Scorpio
rěn dōng téng	忍冬藤	Lonicerae, Caulis
rén shēn	人参	Ginseng, Radix
sān léng	三棱	Sparganii, Rhizoma
sān qī	三七	Notoginseng, Radix
sāng shèn	桑椹	Mori, Fructus
sāng zhī	桑枝	Mori, Ramulus
shā rén	砂仁	Amomi, Fructus
shān yào	山药	Dioscorea, Rhizome
shān zhā	山楂	Crataegi, Fructus
shé chuáng zǐ	蛇床子	Cnidii, Fructus
shēng dì huáng	生地黄	Rehmanniae Glutinosae, Radix
shēng jiāng	生姜	Zingiberis Recens, Rhizoma
shí gāo	石膏	Gypsum Fibrosum
shí jué míng	石决明	Haliotidis, Concha
shí liú pí	石榴皮	Granati, Pericarpium
shú dì huáng	熟地黄	Rehmanniae Preparata, Radix
shuǐ niú jiǎo	水牛角	Bubali, Cornu
shuǐ yáng suān	水杨酸	Salicylic Acid
táo rén	桃仁	Persicae, Semen
tōng cǎo	通草	Tetrapanacis, Medulla
tǔ fú líng	土茯苓	Smilacis Glabrae, Rhizoma
wēi líng xiān	威灵仙	Clematidis, Radix
xī jiǎo	犀角	Rhinoceri, Cornu
xià kū cǎo	夏枯草	Spica Prunellae Vulgaris
xiāng fù	香附	Cyperi, Rhizoma

Pīnyīn	Chinese	Pharmaceutical
xù duàn	续断	Dipsaci, Radix
xuán shēn	玄参	Scrophulariae Ningpoensis, Radix
xuè jié	血竭	Draconis, Sangusis
yán hú suò	延胡索	Cordialis, Rhizoma
yè jiāo téng	夜交藤	Polygoni Multiflori, Caulis
yě jú huā	野菊花	Chrysanthemi Indici, Flos
yě qiáo mài gēn	野荞麦根	Fagopyri Cymosi, Rhizoma
yì mǔ cǎo	益母草	Leonuri, Herba
yì yǐ rén	薏苡仁	Coices, Semen
yù jīn	郁金	Curcumae Radix
zǎo xiū	蚤休	Paridis, Rhizoma
zé lán	泽兰	Lycopi, Herba
zé xiè	泽泻	Alismatis, Rhizoma
zhāng nǎo	樟脑	Camphora
zhēn zhū mǔ	珍珠母	Margaritaferae, Concha
zhì gān cǎo	炙甘草	Glycyrrhizae Preparata, Radix
zhī má yóu	芝麻油	Sesame Oil
zhī mǔ	知母	Anemarrhenae, Rhizoma
zhī zǐ	栀子	Gardeniae, Fructus
zǐ cǎo	紫草	Arnebiae Seu Lithospermi, Radix

Appendix V: Source Text Bibliography

Pīnyīn title	Chinese title	English title	Author (English)	Author (Chinese)	Published
Bèi Jí Qiān Jīn Yào Fāng	备急千金要方	Essential Prescriptions Worth a Thousand in Gold for Every Emergency	Sūn Sīmiǎo	孙思邈	652
Huáng Dì Nèi Jīng	黄帝内经	The Inner Canon of the Yellow Emperor	Unknown	未知	Between the late Warring States period and the Hàn Dynasty
Shí Shān Yī Àn	石山医案	Medical Cases of Wāng Jī	Collected by his students		1551
Tài Píng Huì Mín Hé Jì Jú Fāng	太平惠民和剂局方	Formulary of the Pharmacy Service for Benefiting the People in the Taiping Era	Imperial Medical Bureau	太医局	1107
Wài Kē Dà Chéng	外科大成	Great Compendium of External Medicine	Qí Kūn	祁坤	1665
Wài Kē Jīng Yào	外科精要	Essence of Diagnosis and Treatment of External Diseases	Chén Zìmíng	陈自明	1263
Wài Kē Jīng Yì	外科精义	Treatment of Surgical Diseases	Qí Dézhī	齐德之	1335
Wài Kē Lǐ Lì	外科理例	Exemplars for Applying the Principles of External Medicine	Wāng Jī	汪机	1531
Wài Kē Qǐ Xuán	外科启玄	Profound Insights on External Diseases	Shēn Dǒuyuán	申斗垣	1604
Wài Kē Xīn Fǎ	外科心法	Essential Teachings on External Medicine	Xuē Jǐ	薛己	1742

Pīnyīn title	Chinese title	English title	Author (English)	Author (Chinese)	Published
Wài Kē Zhēn Quán	外科真诠	Personal Experience in *Wài Kē*	Zōu Yuè	邹岳	1838
Wài Kē Zhèng Zhì Quán Shū	外科证治全书	Complete Book of Patterns and Treatments in External Medicine	Xǔ Kèchāng	许克昌	1831
Wài Kē Zhèng Zōng	外科正宗	True Lineage of External Medicine	Chén Shígōng	陈实功	1617
Wài Tái Mì Yào	外台秘要	Arcane Essentials from the Imperial Library	Wáng Tāo	王焘	752
Wàikē Zhèng Zhì Quán Shēng Jí	外科证治全生集	Complete Compendium of Patterns and Treatments in External Medicine	Wáng Wéi Dé	王维德	1740
Wāng Shíshān Yī Shū Bā Zhǒng	汪石山医书八种	Eight Medical Books of Stone Mountain Wang	Wāng Jī	汪机	1522–1633
Wēn Bìng Tiáo Biàn	温病条辨	Systematic Differentiation of Warm Pathogen Diseases	Wú Jū-Tōng (Wú Táng)	吴鞠通 (吴瑭)	1798
Wǔ Shí Èr Bìng Fāng	五十二病方	Prescriptions for Fifty-Two Diseases	Unknown	未知	1065–771 BC
Xiān Shòu Lǐ Shāng Xù Duàn Mì Fāng	仙授理伤续断秘方	Secret Formulas to Manage Trauma and Reconnect Fractures Received from an Immortal	Lìn Dào Rén	蔺道人	c. 846
Xiǎo Pǐn Fāng	小品方	Essay on Formulas	Chén Yánzhī	陈延之	c. 454–473
Yáng Kē Xīn Dé Jí	疡科心得集	Collected Experiences on Treating Sores	Gāo Bǐngjūn	高秉钧	1806
Yī Fāng Jí Jiě	医方集解	Medical Formulas Collected and Analyzed	Wāng Áng	汪昂	1682
Yī Lěi Yuán Róng	医垒元戎	Supreme Commanders of the Medical Ramparts	Wáng Hào Gǔ	王好古	1291
Yī Xué Rù Mén	医学入门	Introduction to Medicine	Lǐ Chān	李梴	1575

Pīnyīn title	Chinese title	English title	Author (English)	Author (Chinese)	Published
Yì Zhěn Yī Dé	疫疹一得	Achievements Regarding Epidemic Rashes	Yú Lín/Yú Shī-Yú	余霖/余师愚	1794
Yī Zōng Jīn Jiàn	医宗金鉴	The Golden Mirror of Ancestral Medicine	Wú Qiān *et al.*	吴谦等	1736–1743
Zhào Bǐng Nán Lín Chuáng Jīng Yàn Jí	赵炳南临床经验集	Zhào Bǐng Nán's Clinical Experience Set	Zhào Bǐng Nán	赵炳南	1975
Zhèng Zhì Zhǔn Shéng	证治准绳	Standard Differentiation of Patterns and Treatments	Wáng Kěntáng	王肯堂	1602
Zhū Bìng Yuán Hóu Lùn	诸病源侯论	General Treatise on the Etiology and Symptomology of Diseases	Cháo Yuánfāng	巢元方	610
		Complete External Therapies of Chinese Drugs	Xú Xiàngcái	徐象才	1998

Index